NON-SMALL CELL LUNG CANCER

NEW INHIBITORY DESIGNER DRUGS APPROVED FOR USE IN ITS TREATMENT

A book in the Modern Medicine Series

Kerry Atkinson MBBS MD DTM&H FRACP FRCP

About this book

The information describing new inhibitory drugs for non-small cell lung cancer is taken from the USA Food and Drug Administration’s Highlights of Prescribing Information for each drug. Additionally, some information is also taken from the FDA’s Full Prescribing Information for each drug. Both these documents are in the public domain. All other text was written by the author. Some text written by the author occurs within the FDA documents: in this case, the text by the author is in italics and the section is in parentheses. All images used in this book are in the public domain and the reason for their being in the public domain is detailed next to each respective image.

Acknowledgements

I would like to acknowledge the help that I received from Jim Severino in designing the covers for this book and for uploading it for me to Kindle Direct Publishing.

Key words: cancer medicine; new drugs for cancer, inhibitory drugs for cancer, tyrosine kinase inhibitors, improvements in cancer treatment

Other books by Kerry Atkinson

Medical books

1. Graft-versus-Host Disease. Editors, S Burakoff, H J Deeg, J Ferrara, K Atkinson. Marcel Dekker Inc, New York, 1990.
2. Clinical Bone Marrow Transplantation. First edition. Editor, K Atkinson. Cambridge University Press, Cambridge UK, 1994.
3. The BMT Data Book: A Manual for Bone Marrow and Blood Stem Cell Transplantation. K. Atkinson, Cambridge University Press, Cambridge UK, 1998.
4. Clinical Bone Marrow and Blood Stem Cell Transplantation. Second Edition. Editor, K. Atkinson. Cambridge University Press, Cambridge UK, 2000.
5. Clinical Bone Marrow and Blood Stem Cell Transplantation. Third Edition. Eds, K. Atkinson, R Champlin, J Ritz, M Brenner, P Ljungman and W Fibbe. Cambridge University Press, Cambridge UK, 2004.
6. The BMT Data Book. Second edition. R Munker, HM Lazarus and K. Atkinson, Cambridge University Press, Cambridge UK, 2009.
7. The BMT Data Book: Including Cellular Therapy. Third edition. R Munker, C Hildebrandt, HM Lazarus and K. Atkinson, Cambridge University Press, Cambridge UK. 2013.
8. Hematopoietic Cell Transplants: Concepts, Controversies and Future Directions. Eds HM Lazarus, RP Gale, A Keating, A Bacigalupo, R Munker, K Atkinson, A Syed. Cambridge University Press, Cambridge, UK. 2017.
9. The Biology and Therapeutic Application of Mesenchymal Cells. Ed. K Atkinson. Wiley/Blackwell. 2017
10. Revolutionizing Tropical Medicine. Eds. K Atkinson and D Mabey. Wiley/Blackwell Publishers Inc. 2019.

11. Asthma: Targeted Biological Treatments 2020. Kindle Direct Publishing, 2020. e-book and paperback
12. Atopic Dermatitis: Targeted Biological Treatments 2020. Kindle Direct Publishing, 2020. e-book and paperback
13. Psoriasis: Targeted Biological Treatments 2020. Kindle Direct Publishing, 2020. e-book and paperback
14. Crohn's disease and ulcerative colitis: Targeted Biological Treatments 2020. Kindle Direct Publishing, 2020. e-book and paperback
15. Rheumatoid arthritis, Juvenile Idiopathic Arthritis, Ankylosing spondylitis, Psoriatic Arthritis and Gout: Targeted Biological Treatments 2020. Kindle Direct Publishing, 2020. e-book and paperback
16. Small Cell Lung Cancer: Targeted Biological Treatments 2020. Kindle Direct Publishing, 2020. e-book and paperback
17. Chronic Myeloid Leukemia: Targeted Biological Treatments 2020. Kindle Direct Publishing, 2020. e-book and paperback
18. Melanoma: Targeted Biological Treatments 2020, Kindle Direct Publishing 2020. e-book and paperback
19. Dementia - A Caregiver's Guide. Kindle Direct Publishing 2020. e-book
20. Breast Cancer: Targeted Biological Treatments 2021. Kindle Direct Publishing 2021. e-book and paperback
21. Non-melanoma Skin Cancers: Targeted Biological and Specifically Designed Therapeutic agents. 2022. Kindle Direct Publishing 2021. e-book and paperback
22. Hodgkin Lymphoma: Targeted Biological Treatments. 2022. Kindle Direct Publishing 2022. e-book and paperback
23. Chimeric Antigen Receptor (CAR) T Cells: The second Revolution in Cellular Therapy. 2022. Kindle Direct Publishing 2022. e-book and paperback
24. Acute lymphoblastic leukemia: targeted immune therapeutic agents. Kindle Direct Publishing 2023. e-book and paperback

25. Artificial Intelligence and Medicine. A book in the Modern Medicine series. Kindle Direct Publishing 2024. e-book and paperback

Natural history/conservation books

26. Bird facts for everyone. K Atkinson. Outskirts Press Inc., Denver, USA. 2014

27. Birds, Birds, Birds. Kindle Direct Publishing 2020. e-book and paperback

28. A Field Guide to the Wild Habitats of Sydney Australia. Kindle Direct Publishing 2021. e-book and paperback

29. Conserving New Zealand's Endangered Species. Kindle Direct Publishing 2021. e-book and paperback

30. Conserving Australia's Endangered Species. Kindle Direct Publishing 2021. e-book and paperback

31. Nature's Wonders: Britain and Ireland. Kindle Direct Publishing 2021. e-book and paperback.

32. Nature's Wonders: Spain and Bulgaria. Kindle Direct Publishing 2022. e-book and paperback.

33. Nature's Wonders: France's Camargue, the Swiss National Park and Portugal. Kindle Direct Publishing 2022. e-book and paperback.

34. Nature's Wonders: Cuba. Kindle Direct Publishing 2022. e-book and paperback.

35. Nature's Wonders: Japan in Winter Kindle Direct Publishing 2022. e-book and paperback.

36. Nature's Wonders: India. Kindle Direct Publishing 2022. e-book and paperback.

37. Nature's Wonders: Tanzania. Kindle Direct Publishing 2022. e-book and paperback.

38. The Silk Road: Uzbekistan and Kazakhstan – A Book in the Nature's Wonders Series. 2022. Kindle Direct Publishing 2022. e-book and paperback.

39. Madagascar – Land of Lemurs and Chameleons: a book in the Nature's Wonders series 2023. Kindle Direct Publishing 2022. e-book and paperback.

40. South Africa - Kalahari to the Cape - a book in the Nature's Wonders series. Kindle Direct Publishing 2022. e-book and paperback

41. Nature's Wonders – Finland - land of owls and lakes. Kindle Direct Publishing 2023. e-book and paperback

42. Nature's Wonders – Ethiopia. Kindle Direct Publishing 2023. e-book and paperback

43. Nature's Wonders – Kakadu National Park and Central Australia. Kindle Direct Publishing 2023. e-book and paperback

44. Nature's Wonders – Lord Howe Island, Australia. Kindle Direct Publishing 2023. e-book and paperback

45. Norway above the Arctic Circle in March. A book in the Nature's Wonders series. Kindle Direct Publishing 2024. e-book and paperback

46. The Inside Passage and the Pribilof Islands. A book in the Nature's Wonders series. Kindle Direct Publishing 2024. e-book and paperback

47. Orca! (and some interesting bird species in Washington State). Kindle Direct Publishing 2024. e-book

Other books

48. Paintings by Kerry Atkinson 2019 – 2021. Kindle Direct Publishing 2021. e-book and paperback.

49. Ferrari Road Cars. Kindle Direct Publishing 2022. e-book and paperback.

50. Paintings by Kerry Atkinson 2022. Kindle Direct Publishing 2022. e-book and paperback.

51. Samuel Beckett and Bob Dylan – living in a Shakespearean era. Kindle Direct Publishing 2022. e-book and paperback.

52. Paintings and sculptures by Kerry Atkinson 2023. Kindle Direct Publishing 2023. e-book and paperback.

53. Ten influential European paintings. Kindle Direct Publishing 2023. e-book and paperback

54. The Pillars of Rock 'N Roll. Kindle Direct Publishing 2024. e-book and paperback

55. Early 20th century western paintings - a smorgasbord of color and radical shapes. Kindle Direct Publishing 2024. e-book and paperback

56. Insects and other wildlife included in Dutch flower paintings from the Dutch golden age. Kindle Direct Publishing 2024. e-book and paperback

Table of Contents

1. Author's preface, page 7
2. Introduction to targeted biologic and specifically designed therapeutic agents, page 9
3. The biology of normal human cells, page 12
4. The biology of malignant human cells, page 28
5. Overview of lung cancer, page 32
6. Overview of the diagnostic work-up and treatment of non-small cell lung cancer, page 34
7. Small inhibitory molecules (tyrosine kinase inhibitors) in the treatment of non-small cell lung cancer, page 40

7.1. Drugs used for drug-sensitizing mutations of the epidermal growth factor receptor (EGFR), page 40

(i) Osimertinib (TAGRISSO), page 40

(ii) Lazertinib (LAZCLUZE), page 52

7.2. Drugs used for drug-sensitizing mutations of the anaplastic lymphoma kinase gene, page 58

(i) Alectinib (ALECENZA), page 58

(ii) Brigatinib (ALUNBERG), page 61

(iii) Lorlatinib (LORBRENA), page 67

8. Conclusions, page 72

9. Abbreviations used, page 73

1. Author's preface

The comprehensive understanding of the biology of normal human cells and that of malignant human cells over the last seven decades has led to the development of a large number of new therapeutic agents. Foremost among the beneficiaries of this is medical oncology. When I trained in medical oncology at the Royal Marsden Hospital from 1972 - 1976 there were six agents available for treating non-small cell lung cancer (NSCLC). All were organic chemicals and were known as cytotoxic chemotherapeutic agents. In four diseases they were very effective – even curative. These diseases were childhood (but not adult) acute lymphoblastic leukemia, advanced Hodgkin lymphoma, testicular carcinoma (even if metastatic to the brain) and choriocarcinoma. However, for the four commonest malignant diseases - carcinoma of the lung, carcinoma of the breast, colo-rectal carcinoma and carcinoma of the prostate – they had little efficacy and many side-effects.
The situation today is quite different with over 100 drugs approved by the USA Food and Drug Administration (FDA) in the United States for therapeutic use in non-small cell lung cancer (NSCLC). Other countries are generally slower than the USA to approve them. One group of drugs designed as a result of the new understanding of carcinogenesis are small inhibitory molecules - tyrosine kinase inhibitors. A number of these are approved by the FDA for the treatment of non-small cell lung cancer, and while not yet curative, they are significantly beneficial and are the focus of this book.
Please note:

i. The text of the FDA HIGHLIGHTS OF PRESCRIBING INFORMATION for the drugs described in detail in this book is taken verbatim from the FDA document specific for the drug described. Additionally, I have included the Mechanism of Action of each drug and the Clinical Trial information of each drug. These latter data are taken verbatim from the FDA FULL PRESCRIBING INFORMATION of each drug. Both the FDA Highlights of Prescribing and the FDA Full Prescribing Information are in the public domain

ii. I have added clinical information throughout the book to give information about some adverse clinical events caused by the drugs described. I have made it clear in each instance that this information is NOT in the FDA documents by putting all such additions in *parentheses* and have put the text in *italics.*

iii. I have also put in bold font some headings in the FDA documents that I think are particularly important for the clinician using these drugs to be aware of.

iv. There are three numbering systems in this book: firstly, that of the Table of Contents, which lists chronologically each major section of the book; secondly, that used in the FDA Highlights of Prescribing document; and thirdly, that used in the FDA Full Prescribing Information document. I have not altered the numbering in the case of the two latter documents. Some sections or subsections were omitted from the full FDA Prescribing Information. Thus, the numbering system within the FDA documents for each of the four drugs described is not always chronological.

v. This book deals only with the most recently FDA-approved tyrosine kinase inhibitors for clinical use in non-small cell lung cancer (NSCLC), as indicated in the Table of contents

2. Introduction to targeted biologic and specifically designed therapeutic agents

The five major biomedical revolutions of the second half of the 20th century are

1. The production of monoclonal antibodies
2. The discovery of DNA and how it, RNA and amino acids make proteins
3. Epigenetics and the posttranslational modification of proteins
4. The discovery of cell signalling pathways

5. The cloning of the human genome

Taken together these discoveries in cellular and molecular biology have revealed to scientists appropriate targets for new drugs and the number that have been produced in the last 30 years, and that are still being produced, has hugely enlarged the therapeutic pharmacopeia, producing treatments - even cures - for diseases that were previously untreatable. The majority of these new treatments have been derived because of much more detailed knowledge about how human cells work. They are therefore known as **biological treatments**, often abbreviated to biologics. An example of a biologic is the monoclonal antibody rituximab which reacts specifically with the CD20 antigen present only on B cells, but with no other targets.

In addition, other agents that react specifically with one, or at most, several, targets are **chemically synthesized**: an example is imatinib, which is specific for the tyrosine kinase (TK) domain in abl (the Abelson proto-oncogene), c-kit and PDGF-R (platelet-derived growth factor receptor). Another example is sonedegib, which inhibits activation of the intracellular Hedgehog signalling pathway.

The inclusion of therapeutic agents is based on their specificity for a given target. For example, interleukin 2 (IL-2) would not be included since it has a range of biological activities including the proliferation of T cells, the generation of T cell cytotoxic responses and the recall of cytotoxic T cell memory. Likewise, interferon-alpha (IFN-α) would not be included since its functions include antiviral activity, antiproliferative activity, NK cell activation, cytokine induction, and interferon-stimulated gene-induction activity. This exclusion applies even though each are made constitutively in the body in response to specific diseases: they are biologic agents, but their targets are broad.

This series of books – one for each disease or disease category - explains what the new treatments are, how they work and how they compare, and interact with, conventional treatment. It is important to state that no book in this series makes specific treatment recommendations for any of the diseases covered: such decisions should be initiated and reviewed by an appropriate medical specialist. Much information on each disease is available free of charge from Wikipedia (wikipedia.org), from postgraduate textbooks on each disease and from UpToDate.com: the latter website gives information for patients and caregivers free of charge but a subscription is required for more detailed information (uptodate.com). Rather, the purpose of this series of books is to give information on newly developed biological and specifically designed treatments and their mechanism of action, enabling hopefully the reader to get a handle on these extensive additions to the medical pharmacopeia. This book deals only with biological targeted agents approved by the USA Food and Drug Administration for the treatment of precursor B cell acute lymphoblastic leukemia.

A distinction is sometimes made between **m**onoclonal **a**nti**b**odie**s** (the **mabs**) as “immunotherapy”, the small specifically designed i**n**h**ib**itory molecule**s** (the **nibs**) and the re**cept**or blocking agent**s** (the **cepts**) – the latter sometimes known as decoy receptors. However, since each category of drug has been developed from the comprehensive knowledge of human cell biology discovered over the past seven decades, and as each drug in each category is exquisitely targeted to a specific epitope on a cell surface protein (the mabs), the inhibition of a specific intracellular enzyme process (the nibs), or the blocking of a specific cell surface receptor (the cepts) I prefer to combine the mabs, the nibs and the cepts in the single category of targeted biological treatments. An example from each category are rituximab, imatinib and etanercept.

A fourth type of biological targeted agents has now been FDA-approved for therapeutic use – sonidegib and vismodegib – both of which specifically target the intracellular **Hedgehog pathway** and are now both FDA-approved for treatment of basal cell carcinoma of the skin.

A fifth type of biological targeted agents approved by the FDA for treatment in a large number of different cancers are the **check point inhibitors**, which decrease the suppression of T cell activity common in all cancers, thus enabling the patients’ own T cells to act against their cancer. These agents have made significant improvements in the outcome of a number of malignancies, notably in malignant melanoma

There is now a sixth type of biological targeted therapeutic agents that have been approved by the FDA for therapeutic use: chimeric antigen receptor modified **(CAR) T cells**. The first such agent – tisagenlecleucel – was approved by the USA FDA in 2017 for use in people with acute lymphoblastic leukemia. CAR T cells are an innovative cellular immunotherapeutic approach that involves genetic modification of autologous T cells such that they express target tumor antigen/s as well as a component of the T cell activation pathway – the CD3 zeta chain. T cell surface glycoprotein CD3 zeta chain, also known as T cell receptor T3 zeta chain or CD247, together with T cell receptor alpha/beta and gamma/delta heterodimers and CD3-gamma, -delta, and -epsilon, forms the T cell receptor-CD3 complex. The zeta chain plays an important role in coupling antigen recognition to several intracellular signal-transduction pathways. Upon recognition of the tumor antigen, the transduced T cells become cytotoxic and destroy the tumor cell.

CAR T cells represent the second type of cellular therapy to be therapeutically successful. The first successful cellular therapy was the use **of hematopoietic stem cells**, introduced in the late 1960s, which offered curative treatment for diseases that were not curable by any other type of therapy.

This new drug discovery phenomenon is a therapeutic tsunami which shows no sign of slowing. The pharmacopeia has increased enormously and all medical students should consider doing a Master's degree or a PhD in molecular biology. It is only by working in a cellular or molecular biology laboratory (usually combined) that one can really understand how each of these new medications work.

It should be noted that all text on each individual drug is taken directly from the USA FDA's Highlights of Prescribing document and the FDA's Full Prescribing Information for that drug, including the drug's generic name, its brand name, the indications for which it is approved, its mechanism of action, and other details on warnings, precautions, adverse events and specific patient populations. Both these documents are in the public domain and can be accessed at https://www.accessdata.fda.gov/scripts/cder/daf/.

All images used are in the public domain. Each image carries the legend written by the creator of the image as well as full attribution details required by the creator.

Examples of inhibitory drugs approved by the FDA for non- malignant diseases and malignant diseases

- Janus kinase inhibitors – eg, tofacitinib in Crohn's disease, ruxolitinib for steroid-refractory acute graft-versus-host disease

- Bruton's tyrosine kinase inhibitor – eg, ibrutinib for chronic graft-versus-host disease
- Other human tyrosine kinase inhibitors – eg, imatinib for systemic mastocytosis

3. The biology of normal human cells

To fully understand how these new therapeutic agents work it is useful to understand how cells work – in particular, what signalling pathways they use. Normal cells and cells in tissues affected by non- diseases use signalling pathways often different from those used by cells. All human cells are derived from a single totipotent stem cell which is produced by the fusion of a single sperm with a single ovum. This totipotent stem cell has all the genes on its chromosomes responsible for the future growth and development of the fetus, including reproductive capacity. Cell biology is concerned with the physiological properties, metabolic processes, signalling pathways, life cycle, chemical composition and interactions of cells with their environment. Cell biology involves genetics, biochemistry, molecular
biology, immunology and cytochemistry. Human cells are eukaryotes - they contain organelles. The generalized structure of a eukaryotic cell is shown in Figure 1.

Figure 1. A diagram of a mammalian cell

This image has been released into the public domain by its author, LadyofHats (Mariana Ruiz). Source: own work using Adobe Illustrator. Image renamed from Image:Animal cell structure.svg.
https://commons.wikimedia.org/wiki/File:Animal_cell_structure_en.svg. No changes have been made to this image.

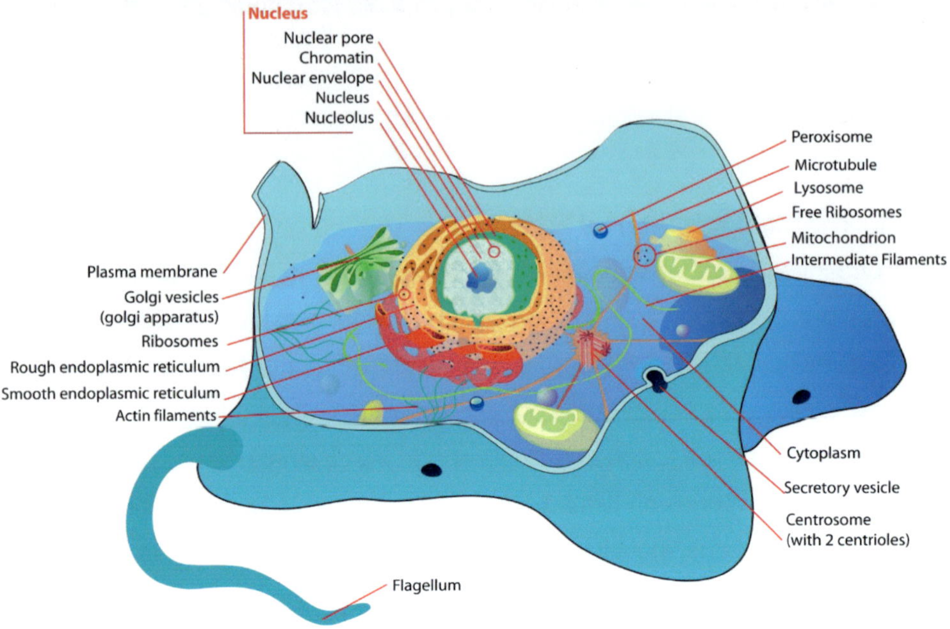

Most of the processes of eukaryotic cells are performed by a mixture of small organic molecules, inorganic ions, hormones and water. Approximately 75-85% of the cell's volume is due to water making it an indispensable solvent as a result of its polarity and structure. The shape of cells are generally round and spherical or oval.

The main constituents of the cell include proteins and lipids which are either free-flowing or membrane-bound, along with different internal compartments known as organelles. The cytoplasm is all of the material within a cell, enclosed by the cell membrane, except for the cell nucleus. The material inside the nucleus and contained within the nuclear membrane is termed the nucleoplasm. A cell's DNA, contained on the cell's chromosomes, is located within the cell's nucleus. The main components of the cytoplasm are cytosol – a gel-like substance, the organelles – the cell's internal sub-structures - and various cytoplasmic inclusions. Cell are composed of hydrophilic and hydrophobic regions. The hydrophilic regions of the cell are on both the inside and outside of the cell, while the hydrophobic regions are within the phospholipid bilayer of the cell membrane. A diagram of a mammalian cell membrane is shown in Figure 2. This shows the detailed diagram of lipid bilayer cell membrane. The cell membrane, also called the plasma membrane or plasmalemma, biological molecules, primarily proteins and lipids, which are involved in a vast array of cellular processes. It also serves as the attachment point for both the intracellular cytoskeleton and, if present, the cell wall.

Figure 2.

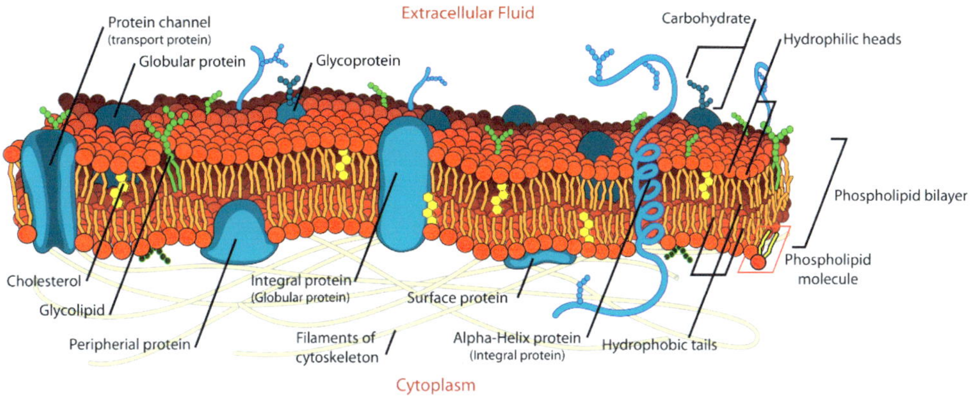

This image has been released into the public domain by its author, LadyofHats (Mariana Ruiz). Source: Own work. Image renamed from File:Cell membrane detailed diagram.svg. https://commons.wikimedia.org/wiki/File:Cell_membrane_detailed_diagram_en.svg. No changes have been made to this image.

In order for molecules to participate in reactions within the cell, they need to be able to cross this membrane layer to get into the cell. They accomplish this process of gaining access to the cell via osmotic pressure, diffusion, concentration gradients, and membrane channels. Inside the cell are extensive internal suB cellular membrane-bounded compartments called organelles.

Figure 3. Some of the cell surface proteins and internal signalling pathways of a normal human cell.

This image is in the public domain in the United States because it is a work prepared by an officer or employee of the United States Government as part of that person's official duties under the terms of Title 17, Chapter 1, Section 105 of the US Code. Source: http://dir.niehs.nih.gov/dirlst/imagemap/cell.jpg. https://commons.wikimedia.org/wiki/File:NIEHScell.jpg. No changes have been made to this image.

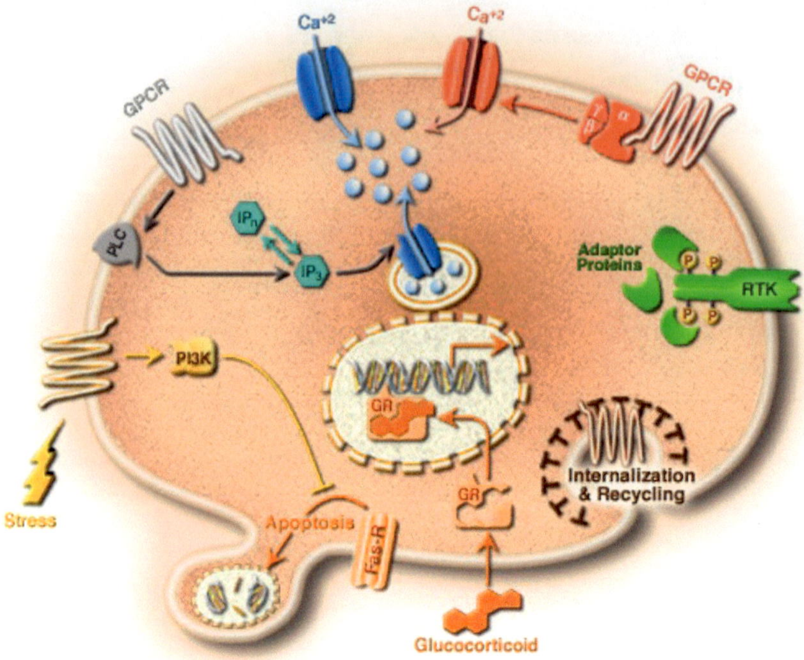

Cell growth pertains to the increase in the number of cells present in an organism as it grows and develops; in order for the organism to grow the number of cells present must increase. To enable cell growth and development the cell goes through the steps of the cell cycle: DNA replication, cell division, regeneration, specialization, and cell death. The cell cycle is divided into four distinct phases, G1, S, G2, and M. The G phases (cell growth) make up approximately 95% of the cycle. After proliferation cells then differentiate to become specialized in order to form specialized tissues, then organs and ultimately systems. The G phases along with the S phase – DNA replication, damage and repair - are considered to be the interphase portion of the cycle. While the M phase (mitosis and cytokinesis) is the cell division portion of the cycle. The cell cycle is regulated by a series of signalling factors and complexes such as cyclin-dependent kinases and p53. When the cell has completed its growth process, and if it is found to be damaged or altered, it undergoes cell death, either by apoptosis or necrosis, in order to eliminate the threat it can cause to the organism's survival. Some of the main cell surface proteins and internal signalling processes are shown in Figure 3.

Essential cell processes include

- Active transport and passive transport – the movement of molecules into and out of cells
- Adhesion - holding cells and tissues together
- Cell movement - chemotaxis, contraction and cilia
- Cell signalling - regulation of cell behaviour by signals from outside and inside the cell
- Division – the process by which cells reproduce either by mitosis (to produce clones of the parent cell) or meiosis (to produce haploid gametes either male [sperm)] or female [ova]) dependent on the gender of the organism
- DNA repair - cell death and cell senescence
- Metabolism - glycolysis, respiration, photosynthesis, and chemosynthesis
- Signal transduction - the process by which the activities in the cell are regulated
- Transcription and mRNA splicing - gene expression

Three of the most important processes – signal transduction, gene expression and apoptosis (also known as programmed cell death) - are described furtherl below. Some of the most important pathways for understanding the basis of targeted therapies, such as the pathways for angiogenesis, interleukin (IL) 4, IL-12 and IL-23 and the TNF pathways are described in chapters dealing with the therapeutic use of molecules involved in these pathways.

Signal transduction and cell signalling pathways

Signal transduction is the process by which a chemical or physical signal is transmitted through a cell as a series of molecular events, most commonly protein phosphorylation catalysed by protein kinases, which ultimately results in a cellular response. Proteins responsible for detecting stimuli such as ligands are termed receptors The changes elicited by ligand binding to a receptor give rise to a biochemical cascade otherwise known as a signalling path.

When signalling pathways interact with one another they form networks, which allow cellular responses to be coordinated, often by combinatorial signalling events. At the molecular level, such responses include changes in the transcription or translation of genes, and post-translational and conformational changes in proteins, as well as changes in their location. These molecular events are the basic mechanisms controlling cell growth, proliferation, metabolism and many other processes. In multicellular organisms, signal transduction pathways have evolved to regulate cell communication in a wide variety of ways.

Each component (or node) of a signalling pathway is classified according to the role it plays with respect to the initial stimulus. Ligands are termed first messengers, while receptors are the signal transducers, which then activate primary effectors. Such effectors are often linked to second messengers, which can activate secondary effectors, and so on. Depending on the efficiency of the nodes, a signal can be amplified (a concept known as signal gain), so that one signalling molecule can generate a response involving hundreds to millions of molecules With the advent of computational biology, the analysis of signalling pathways and networks has become an essential tool to understand cellular functions and disease, including signalling rewiring mechanisms underlying responses to acquired drug resistance.

Ligands

The majority of signal transduction pathways involve the binding of signalling molecules, known as ligands, to receptors that trigger events inside the cell. The binding of a signalling molecule with a receptor causes a change in the conformation of the receptor, known as receptor activation. Most ligands are soluble molecules from the extracellular medium which bind to cell surface receptors. These include growth factors, cytokines and neurotransmitters. Components of the extracellular matrix such as fibronectin and hyaluronan can also bind to such receptors (integrins and CD44, respectively). In addition, some molecules such as steroid hormones are lipid-soluble and thus cross the plasma membrane to reach nuclear receptors.

Some receptors such as HER2/neu are capable of ligand-independent activation when overexpressed or mutated. This leads to constitutive activation of the pathway, which may or may not be overturned by compensation mechanisms. In the case of HER2, which acts as a dimerization partner of other EGFRs, constitutive activation leads to hyperproliferation and cancer – primarily some cases of breast cancer and gastric cancer (HER2/neu is also known as receptor tyrosine-protein kinase erbB-2, CD340, proto-oncogene Neu and ERBB2). A ribbon diagram of the Fab fragment of trastuzumab, a monoclonal antibody, bound to the extracellular domain of HER2 is shown in Figure 4.

Figure 4. A ribbon diagram of the Fab fragment of trastuzumab

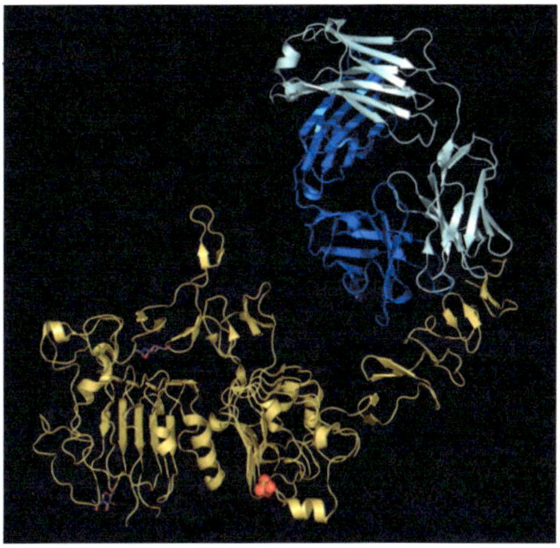

Ribbon diagram of the Fab fragment of trastuzumab, a monoclonal antibody, bound to the extracellular domain of HER2. Legend: Trastuzumab Fab fragment, heavy chain ; Trastuzumab Fab fragment, light chain ; HER2, extracellular domain

This image is in the public domain because its creator, Fvasconcellos, has placed it there. https://commons.wikimedia.org/wiki/File:Trastuzumab_Fab-HER2_complex_1N8Z.png#/media/File:Trastuzumab_Fab-HER2_complex_1N8Z.png; https://commons.wikimedia.org/wiki/User:Fvasconcellos. Created using Accelrys DS Visualizer Pro 1.6 and GIMP. More information: Cho HS, Mason K, Ramyar KX, et al. (2003). "Structure of the extracellular region of HER2 alone and in complex with the Herceptin Fab". Nature 421 (6924): 756–60. PMID 12610629. doi:10.1038/nature01392. No changes have been made to this image.

Extracellular receptors, ligand binding, messengers and adaptor proteins

Extracellular receptors are integral transmembrane proteins that span the plasma membrane of the cell, with one part of the receptor on the outside of the cell and the other on the inside. Signal transduction occurs as a result of a ligand binding to the outside region of the receptor (the ligand does not pass through the membrane). Ligand-receptor binding induces a change in the conformation of the inside part of the receptor, a process sometimes called "receptor activation". This results in either the activation of an enzyme domain of the receptor or the exposure of a binding site for other intracellular signalling proteins within the cell, eventually propagating the signal through the cytoplasm.

In mammalian cells most intracellular proteins activated by a ligand/receptor interaction possess an enzymatic activity; examples include tyrosine kinases and phosphatases. Often such enzymes are covalently linked to the receptor. Some of them create second messengers such as cyclic AMP and IP3, the latter controlling the release of intracellular calcium stores into the cytoplasm. Other activated proteins interact with adaptor proteins that facilitate signalling protein interactions and coordination of signalling complexes necessary to respond to a particular stimulus. Enzymes and adaptor proteins are both responsive to various second messenger molecules.

Many adaptor proteins and enzymes activated as part of signal transduction possess specialized protein domains that bind to specific secondary messenger molecules. For example, calcium ions bind to the EF hand domains of calmodulin, allowing it to bind and activate calmodulin-dependent kinase.

The following major extracellular receptor/ligand binding pathways will be discussed in more detail below:

- G protein-coupled receptors
- Tyrosine, seronine/threonine- and histidine-specific protein kinases
- Integrins
- Toll-like receptors
- Ligand-gated ion binding channels

G proteins, also known as guanine nucleotide-binding proteins, are a family of proteins that act as molecular switches inside cells, and are involved in transmitting signals from a variety of stimuli outside a cell to its interior. Their activity is regulated by factors that control their ability to bind to and hydrolyze guanosine triphosphate (GTP) to guanosine diphosphate (GDP). When they are bound to GTP, they are 'on', and, when they are bound to GDP, they are 'off'.

They possess seven transmembrane domains and are linked to a heterotrimeric G protein. A ribbon diagram of a G protein is shown in Figure 6. Beta and gamma subunits of G-protein are shown by blue and red, respectively, in the phosducin transducin beta-gamma complex. (Phosducin binds tightly to the beta gamma subunits (Gt beta gamma) of the heterotrimeric G protein transducin, preventing Gt beta gamma reassociation with Gt alpha-GDP and thereby inhibiting the G-protein cycle).

Figure 6. Ribbon diagram of a G protein

This image has been released into the public domain by its creator, Andrei Lomize, has placed it there. By Andrei Lomize - Own work, Public Domain,

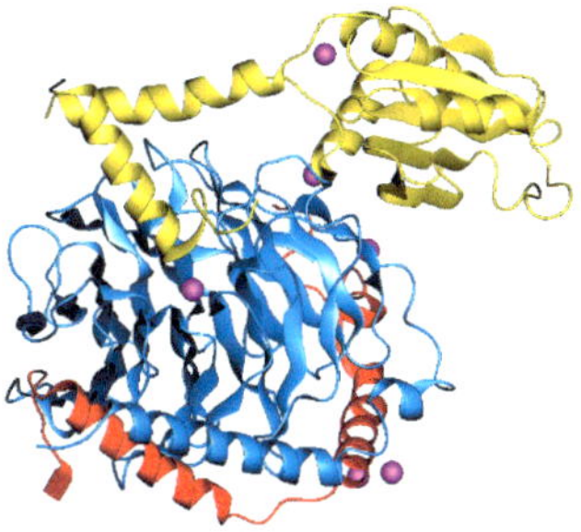

Tyrosine and seronine/threonine-specific protein kinases

Receptor tyrosine kinases (RTKs) are transmembrane proteins with an intracellular kinase domain and an extracellular domain that binds ligands; examples include growth factor receptors such as the insulin receptor. To perform signal transduction, RTKs need to form dimers in the plasma membrane. The dimer is stabilized by ligands binding to the receptor. The interaction between the cytoplasmic domains stimulates the autophosphorylation of tyrosine residues within the intracellular kinase domains of the RTKs, causing conformational changes. Subsequent to this, the receptors' kinase domains are activated, initiating phosphorylation signaling cascades of downstream cytoplasmic molecules that facilitate various cellular processes such as cell differentiation and metabolism. Many serine/threonine and dual-specificity protein kinases are important for signal transduction, either acting downstream of receptor tyrosine kinases, or as membrane-embedded or cell-soluble versions in their own right. The process of signal transduction involves around 560 known protein kinases and pseudokinanases, encoded by the human kinome. The kinome of an organism is the complete set of protein kinases encoded in its genome.

As is the case with GPCRs, proteins that bind GTP play a major role in signal transduction from the activated RTK into the cell. In this case, the G proteins are members of the Ras, Rho, and Raf families, referred to collectively as small G proteins. They act as molecular switches usually tethered to membranes by isoprenyl groups linked to their carboxyl ends. Upon activation, they assign proteins to specific membrane subdomains where they participate in signalling. Activated RTKs in turn activate small G proteins that activate guanine nucleotide exchange factors such as SOS1. Once activated, these exchange factors can activate more small G proteins, thus amplifying the receptor's initial signal. The mutation of certain RTK genes, as with that of GPCRs, can result in the expression of receptors that exist in a constitutively activated state. Such mutated genes may act as oncogenes. An example is the BCR-ABL gene, which is translated to the BCR-ABL protein, a growth factor responsible for the development of chronic myeloid leukemia (CML). The first tyrosine kinase inhibitor developed that was therapeutically successful is imatinib, now routinely used as first-line treatment of CML, obviating the need in many cases of the only curative treatment for CML – allogeneic hematopoietic stem cell transplantaion, a procedure that had a treatment-related mortality of 20-30%.

Integrins

Integrins are produced by a wide variety of cells. They play a role in cell attachment to other cells and the extracellular matrix and in the transduction of signals from extracellular matrix components such as fibronectin and collagen (Figure 7).

Figure 7. An overview of integrin-mediated signal transduction, adapted from Hehlgens et al. (2007).

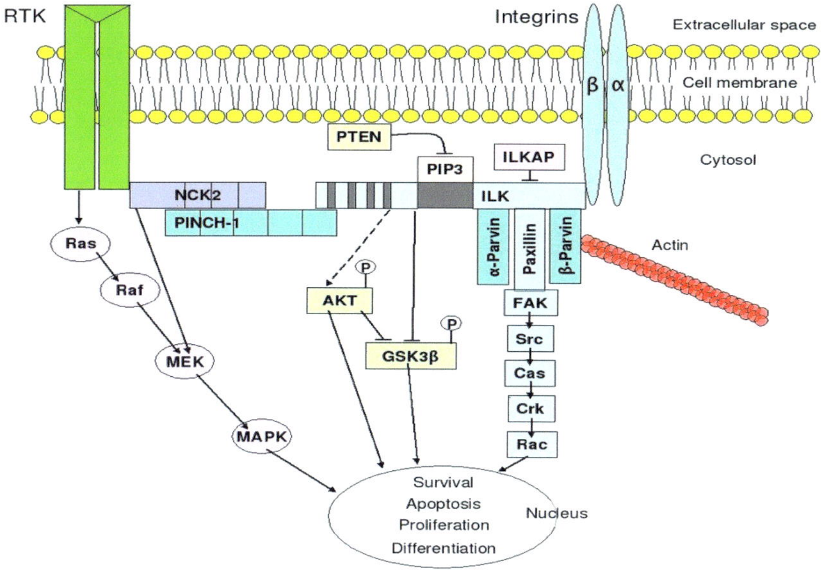

This image has been released into the public domain by its author, K.murphy at English Wikipedia. https://commons.wikimedia.org/wiki/File:Integrin_sig_trans_overview.jpeg. Original source: Hehlgans S, Haase M, Cordes N (Jan 2007). "Signalling via integrins: implications for cell survival and anticancer strategies". Biochimica et Biophysica Acta. 1775 (1): 163–80. doi:10.1016/j.bbcan.2006.09.001. PMID 17084981.

Ligand binding to the extracellular domain of integrins changes the protein's conformation, clustering it at the cell membrane to initiate signal transduction. Integrins lack kinase activity; hence, integrin-mediated signal transduction is achieved through a variety of intracellular protein kinases and adaptor molecules, the main coordinator being integrin-linked kinase. As shown in Figure 7, cooperative integrin-RTK signaling determines the timing of cellular survival, apoptosis, proliferation and differentiation.

Toll-like receptors

When activated, toll-like receptors (TLRs) take adapter molecules within the cytoplasm of cells in order to propagate a signal.

Four adaptor molecules are known to be involved in signalling. These are Myd88, TIRAP, TRIF, and TRAM. These adapter molecules activate other intracellular molecules such as IRAK1, IRAK4, TBK1, and IKKi that amplify the signal, eventually leading to the induction or suppression of genes that cause certain responses. Thousands of genes are activated by TLR signalling, implying that this method constitutes an important gateway for gene modulation.

Messenger systems

First messengers are the signalling molecules (hormones, neurotransmitters and paracrine/autocrine agents) that reach the cell from the extracellular fluid and bind to their specific receptors.

Second messengers are the substances that enter the cytoplasm and act within the cell to trigger a response. Second messengers serve as chemical relays from the plasma membrane to the cytoplasm, thus carrying out intracellular signal transduction.

Calcium

The release of calcium ions from the endoplasmic reticulum into the cytosol results in its binding to signalling proteins that are then activated. It is then sequestered in the smooth endoplasmic reticulum and the mitochondria. Calcium is used in many processes including muscle contraction, neurotransmitter release from nerve endings, and cell migration. The three main pathways that lead to its activation are GPCR pathways, RTK pathways, and gated ion channels. It regulates proteins either directly or by binding to an enzyme.

Cellular responses

Gene activations and metabolism alterations are examples of cellular responses to extracellular stimulation that require signal transduction. Gene activation leads to further cellular effects, since the products of responding genes include instigators of activation. Transcription factors produced as a result of a signal transduction cascade can activate even more genes. Hence, an initial stimulus can trigger the expression of a large number of genes, leading to physiological events. Examples are the increased uptake of glucose from the blood stream and the migration of neutrophils to sites of infection.

Mammalian cells require stimulation for cell division and survival. In the absence of growth factor, apoptosis (programmed cell death – see below) ensues. Such requirements for extracellular stimulation are necessary for controlling cell behavior. Signal transduction pathways are perceived to be so central to biological processes that a large number of diseases are attributed to their dysregulation. Three basic types of signals determine cellular growth:

1. **Stimulatory signals (growth factors)**

Transcription-dependent response
Steroids are an example of this. They bind DNA, which needs to be transcribed. The produced mRNA needs to be translated, and the produced protein/peptide can undergo posttranslational modification (PMT).

Transcription-independent response
Epidermal growth factor (EGF) is an example. It binds to the epidermal growth factor receptor (EGFR), which causes dimerization and autophosphorylation of the EGFR, which in turn activates the intracellular signalling pathway.

2. **Inhibitory signals (cell-cell contact)**

3. **Permissive signals (cell-matrix interactions)**

The combination of these signals are integrated in an altered cytoplasmic machinery which leads to altered cell behaviour.

Major cell signalling pathways
The following are some of the major cell signalling pathways, demonstrating how ligands binding to their receptors can affect second messengers and eventually result in altered cellular responses.

- MAPK/ERK pathway: a pathway that couples intracellular responses to the binding of growth factors to cell surface receptors. This pathway is very complex and includes many protein components. In many cell types, activation of this pathway promotes cell division, and many forms of cancer are associated with aberrations in it.

- cAMP-dependent pathway: cAMP works by activating protein kinase A (PKA, cAMP-dependent protein kinase. Further effects depend mainly on cAMP-dependent protein kinase, which vary based on the type of cell involved.

- IP3/DAG pathway: PLC cleaves the phospholipid phosphatidylinositol 4,5-bisphosphate (PIP2), yielding diacyl glycerol (DAG) and inositol 1,4,5-

triphosphate (IP3). DAG remains bound to the membrane, and IP3 is released as a soluble structure into the cytosol. IP3 then diffuses through the cytosol to bind to IP3 receptors, particular calcium channels in the endoplasmic reticulum (ER). These channels are specific to calcium and allow the passage of only calcium to move through. This causes the cytosolic concentration of calcium to increase, in turn precipitating a cascade of intracellular changes and activity. In addition, calcium and DAG together work to activate PKC, which then phosphorylates other molecules, leading to altered cellular activity.

DNA, RNA and genes

DNA is a molecule composed of two chains that coil around each other to form a double helix carrying the genetic instructions used in the growth, development, functioning, and reproduction of all known organisms and many viruses. DNA and ribonucleic acid (RNA) are nucleic acids. Nucleic acids, together with proteins, lipids and complex carbohydrates (polysaccharides), are one of the four major types of macromolecules that are essential for all known forms of life.

The two DNA strands are also known as polynucleotides as they are composed of simpler monomeric units called nucleotides. Each nucleotide is composed of one of four nitrogen-containing nucleobases (cytosine [C], guanine [G], adenine [A] or thymine [T]), a sugar called deoxyribose, and a phosphate group.

Figure 8 is a graphic of DNA replication. The nitrogenous bases of the two separate polynucleotide strands are bound together, according to base pairing rules (A with T and C with G), with hydrogen bonds to make double-stranded DNA in a helical form.

Figure 8. A graphic of DNA replication.

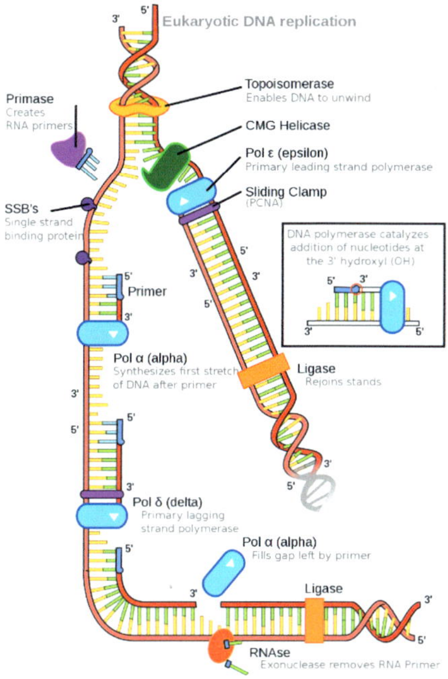

Genes

A gene is a sequence of nucleotides in DNA or RNA that codes for a molecule that has a function. Genes are contained on the chromosomes in the cell nucleus. During gene expression, the DNA is first copied into RNA. The RNA can be directly functional or be the intermediate template for a protein that performs a function. A chromosome consists of a long strand of DNA containing many genes. A human chromosome can have up to 500 million base pairs of DNA with thousands of genes. Gene expression is the process by which information from a gene is used in the synthesis of a functional gene product. These products are often proteins, When the end-product is a protein, genes are first transcribed into RNA, and this transcript is then translated into protein. Several steps in the gene expression process may be modulated, including transcription, RNA splicing, translation and post-translational modification of the protein. Gene regulation gives the cell control over structure and function, and is the basis for cellular differentiation, morphogenesis and the versatility and adaptability of any organism.

Genes are expressed by being transcribed into RNA, and this transcript may then be translated into protein.

Figure 9. Diagram showing how translation of messenger RNA and protein synthesis takes place in ribosomes.

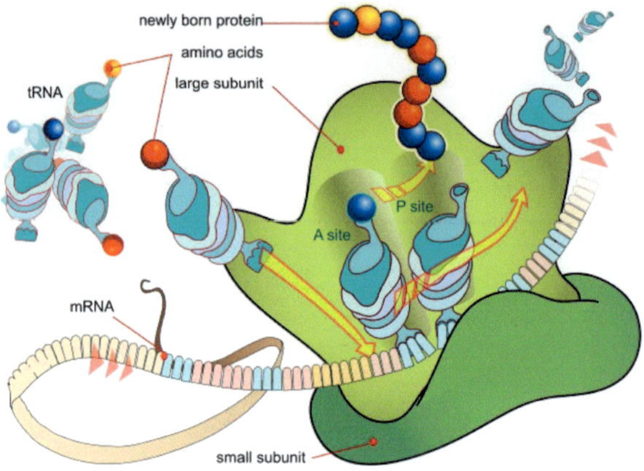

Figure 2. This work has been released into the public domain by its author, LadyofHats. By LadyofHats - Own work based on:[1], [2], [3], [4], [5], [6], [7], and [8]., Public Domain, https://commons.wikimedia.org/w/index.php?curid=4889777; https://en.wikipedia.org/wiki/Translation_(biology)#/media/File:Ribosome_mRNA_translation_en.svg. No changes have been made to this image.

Protein folding

A polypeptide (protein) folds into its characteristic and functional three-dimensional structure from a random coil. Each protein exists as an unfolded polypeptide or random coil when translated from a sequence of messenger (m) RNA into a linear chain of amino acids (Figure 10, left hand image). Amino acids interact with each other to produce a well-defined three-dimensional structure.

Figure 10 shows a protein before (left) and after (right) folding

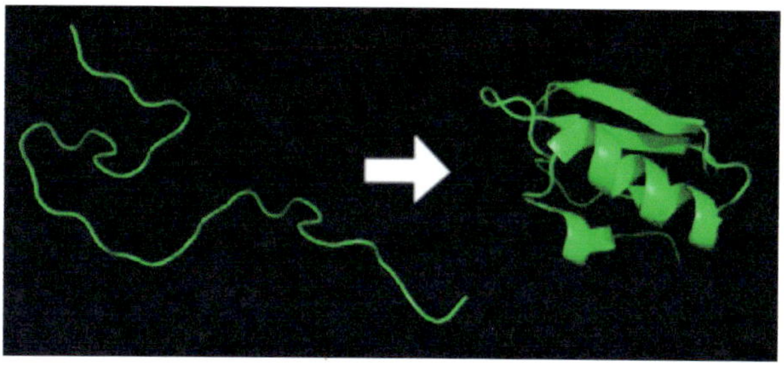

This image, reproduced here from Wikimedia Commons, is in the public domain because its creator has placed it there. By No machine-readable author provided. Dr Kjaergaard assumed (based on copyright claims). - No machine-readable source provided. Own work assumed (based on copyright claims). Public Domain, https://commons.wikimedia.org/w/index.php?curid=1967109. https://en.wikipedia.org/wiki/Protein_folding#/media/File:Protein_folding.png. No changes have been made to this image.

4. The biology of malignant human cells.

Defects in genes (DNA), epigenetic factors and mismatch repair systems can all cause human cells to become malignant.

Genes

With the exception of congenital disorders, malignant human cells have an abnormality of their genetic systems, and differ in this regard to abnormal, but non-malignant, as well as to normal human cells. Carcinogenesis is the formation of a cancer, whereby normal cells are transformed into cancer cells. The process is characterized by changes at the cellular, genetic, and epigenetic levels and abnormal cell division. Cell division is a physiological process that occurs in almost all tissues and under a variety of circumstances. Normally the balance between proliferation and programmed cell death, in the form of apoptosis, is maintained to ensure the integrity of tissues and organs. According to the prevailing accepted theory of carcinogenesis, the somatic mutation
theory, mutations in DNA and epimutations that lead to cancer disrupt these orderly processes by disrupting the programming regulating the processes, upsetting the normal balance between proliferation and cell death. This results in uncontrolled cell division and the evolution of those cells by natural selection in the body. Only certain mutations lead to cancer whereas the majority of mutations do not.

A series of several mutations to certain classes of genes is usually required before a normal cell will transform into a malignant cell.

In order for a normal cell to transform into a malignant cell, the genes that regulate cell growth and differentiation must be altered.

The affected genes are divided into two broad categories. Oncogenes are genes that promote cell growth and reproduction. Tumor suppressor genes are genes that inhibit cell division and survival. Malignant transformation can occur through the formation of novel oncogenes, the inappropriate over-expression of normal oncogenes, or by the under-expression or disabling of tumor suppressor genes. Typically, changes in multiple genes are required to transform a normal cell into a cancer cell (Figure 11)

Figure 11 illustrates that cancers are caused by a series of mutations. Each mutation alters the behavior of the cell to some extent.

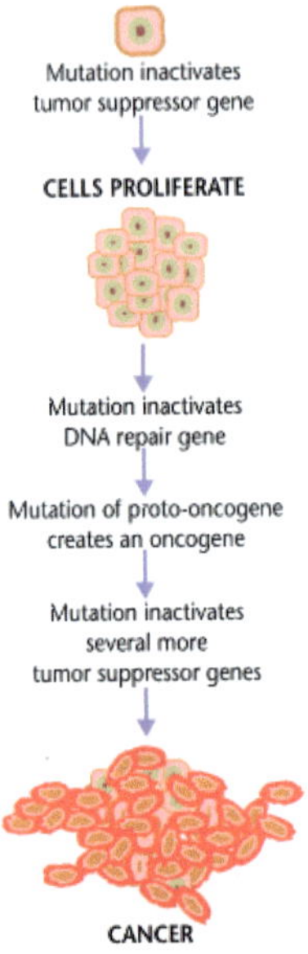

This image is in the public domain because it is a work prepared by an officer or employee of the United States Government as part of that person's official duties under the terms of Title 17, Chapter 1, Section 105 of the US Code. By National Cancer Institute, Public Domain, https://commons.wikimedia.org/w/index.php?curid=1972023. No changes have been made to this image.

The abnormal biological properties of human malignant cells can be summarized as follows:

- Acquisition of self-sufficiency in growth signals, leading to unchecked growth.

- Loss of sensitivity to anti-growth signals, also leading to unchecked growth.
- Loss of capacity for apoptosis, allowing growth despite genetic errors and external anti-growth signals.
- Loss of capacity for senescence, leading to limitless replicative potential (immortality).
- Acquisition of sustained angiogenesis, allowing the tumor to grow beyond the limitations of passive nutrient diffusion.
- Acquisition of ability to invade neighbouring tissues, the defining property of invasive carcinoma.
- Acquisition of ability to seed metastases at distant sites, a late-appearing property of some malignant tumors (carcinomas or others).

Involved in these steps is

- Loss of capacity to repair genetic errors, leading to an increased mutation rate (genomic instability), thus accelerating all the above changes.

Often, the multiple genetic changes that result in cancer may take many years to accumulate. During this time, the biological behavior of the pre-malignant cells slowly changes from the properties of normal cells to those with cancer-like properties (Figure 12).

Figure 12. Tissue can be organized in a continuous spectrum from normal to malignant.

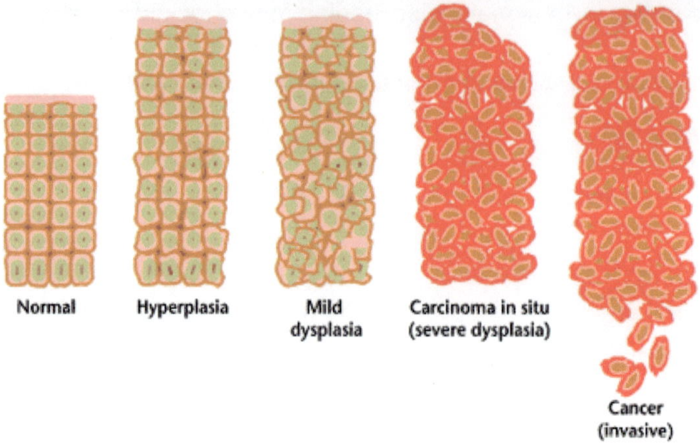

Epigenetic factors also plays a major role in the development of human cancers.

Epigenetic modifications to the DNA of cancer cells do not involve a change in the nucleotide sequence, but instead involve a change in the way the genetic code is expressed. Epigenetic alterations may be just as important, or even more important, than genetic mutations in a cell's transformation to malignancy. In malignant cells loss of expression of genes occurs about 10 times more frequently by transcription silencing (caused by epigenetic promoter hypermethylation of CpG islands) than by mutations. In different types of cancer, a variety of epigenetic mechanisms can be perturbed, such as silencing of tumor suppressor genes and activation of oncogenes by altered CpG island methylation patterns, histone modifications, and dysregulation of DNA-binding proteins.

DNA mismatch repair systems

If DNA repair is deficient, DNA damage tends to accumulate. Such excess DNA damage can increase mutational errors during DNA replication. Excess DNA damage can also increase epigenetic alterations due to errors during DNA repair. Such mutations and epigenetic alterations can give rise to malignancy. Germ line mutations in DNA repair genes cause only 2–5% of colon cancer cases. However, altered expression of microRNAs, causing DNA repair deficiencies, are frequently associated with cancers and may be an important causal factor for such cancers.

In non-hereditary cancers, a deficiency in DNA repair is occasionally found to be due to a mutation in a DNA repair gene, but reduced or absent expression of DNA repair genes is much more frequently due to epigenetic alterations that reduce or silence gene expression.

Cancer therapy procedures such as chemotherapy and radiotherapy work by overwhelming the capacity of the malignant cells to repair DNA damage, resulting in their death. Cells that are most rapidly dividing – most typically cancer cells – are preferentially affected. An important side-effect is that other non-cancerous but rapidly dividing cells such as progenitor cells in the gut, skin, and hematopoietic system are also affected. Modern cancer treatments attempt to localize the DNA damage to cells and tissues only associated with cancer, either by physical means (concentrating the therapeutic agent in the region of the tumor) or by biochemical means (exploiting a feature unique to cancer cells in the body).

5. Overview of lung cancer

There are two types of lung cancer. Non-small cell lung cancer (NSCLC) accounts for 85 % of primary lung cancers. NSCLC is further divided into three histological subtypes – squamous cell lung cancer, adenocarcinoma of the lung and large cell lung cancer. However, their diagnostic work-up and treatment are the same, hence the all-embracing term – non-small cell lung cancer. NSCLC is treatable but not usually curable. One exception to this is a single primary NSCLC tumor with no evidence of secondary spread. This can be cured by surgical resection in a proportion of cases.

The other type of primary lung cancer is small cell lung cancer – accounting for 15% of all primary lung cancers. The is a more aggressive form of lung cancer than NSCLC and is almost always fatal.

Smoking is the biggest risk factor for lung cancer, but 25% of people who get lung cancer have never smoked.

Another other type of malignant disease in the lungs is metastases from a cancer elsewhere in the body – often from thyroid cancer or renal carcinoma. Rarely, some benign lesions are detected in the lungs such as a hamartoma.

The treatment of NSCLC has improved recently due to the availability of three designed small molecular drugs that interfere with the biology of NSCLC cells. They are the topic of this book.

Figure X. The different types of lung cancer and the impact of smoking in their causation

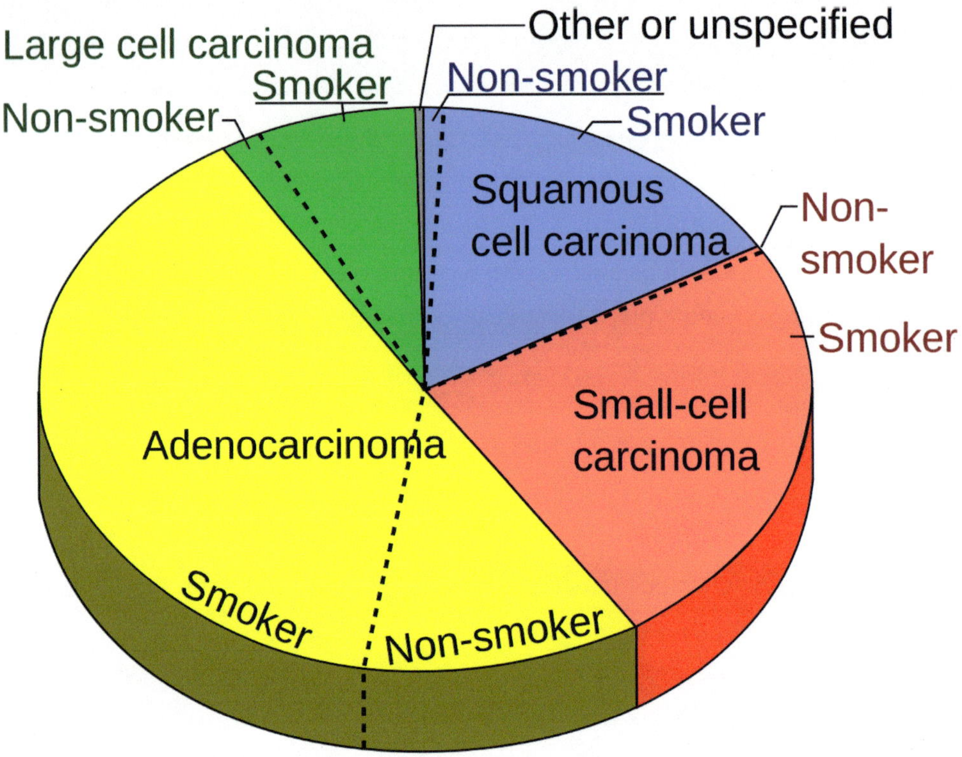

This image is by Mikael Häggström. - Own work, CC0, https://commons.wikimedia.org/w/index.php?curid=15469615; en.wikipedia.org/wiki/Non-small-cell_lung_cancer#/media/File:Pie_chart_of_lung_cancers.svg. This file is made available under the Creative Commons CC0 1.0 Universal Public Domain Dedication. No changes were made to this image.

6. Overview of the diagnostic work-up and treatment of non-small cell lung cancer

The key investigations for NSCLC are a computed tomography (CT) (which uses x-rays) and a positron emission tomography scan (PET) scan (which uses radioactive glucose to determine areas of high metabolism). The CT scan gives much better anatomical detail than a chest x-ray. The PET scan can give additional information regarding the extent of the disease: for example, a CT scan may not detect early involvement of intrathoracic lymph nodes, but a PET scan can do this and the disease may thus be significantly upstaged, often resulting in a change in treatment approach. A bone scan is also often incorporated into the diagnostic evaluation, given the propensity of lung cancers to metastasize to bone.

Figure X. CT scan showing a rounded opacity in the left upper lung (purple arrow) – most likely a primary lung cancer

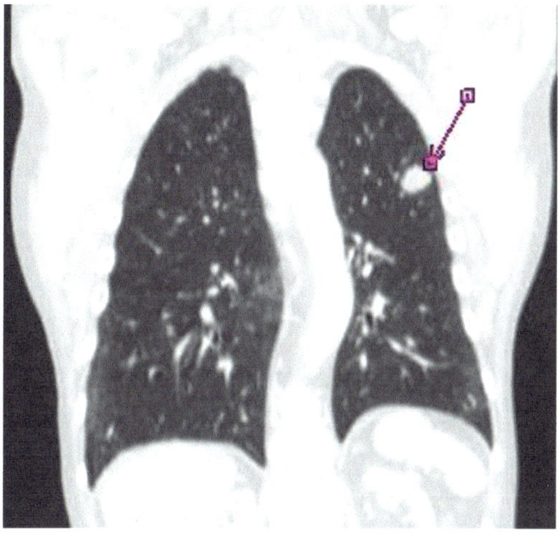

This image is by Lange123 at German Wikipedia - Selbst erstellt: Lange123, 10. Nov. 2004, Public Domain, https://commons.wikimedia.org/w/index.php?curid=12239420; ommons.wikimedia.org/wiki/Category:CT_images_of_cancers_of_bronchus_and_lung#/media/File:Thorax_CT_cor_MPR_peripheres_Bronchialcarcinom_li_OF.jpg. This work has been released into the public domain by its author, Lange123 at German Wikipedia. No changes were made to this image.

One a possible lung cancer has been identified on CT/PET scanning, it is essential to obtain a tissue diagnosis – most commonly by biopsy at bronchoscopy.

Figure X. Photograph of a squamous cell carcinoma of the lung. The tumour is the white tissue in the left middle area of the photograph and is obstructing the bronchus. Beyond and to the right of the tumor tissue, the bronchus is inflamed and contains mucus.

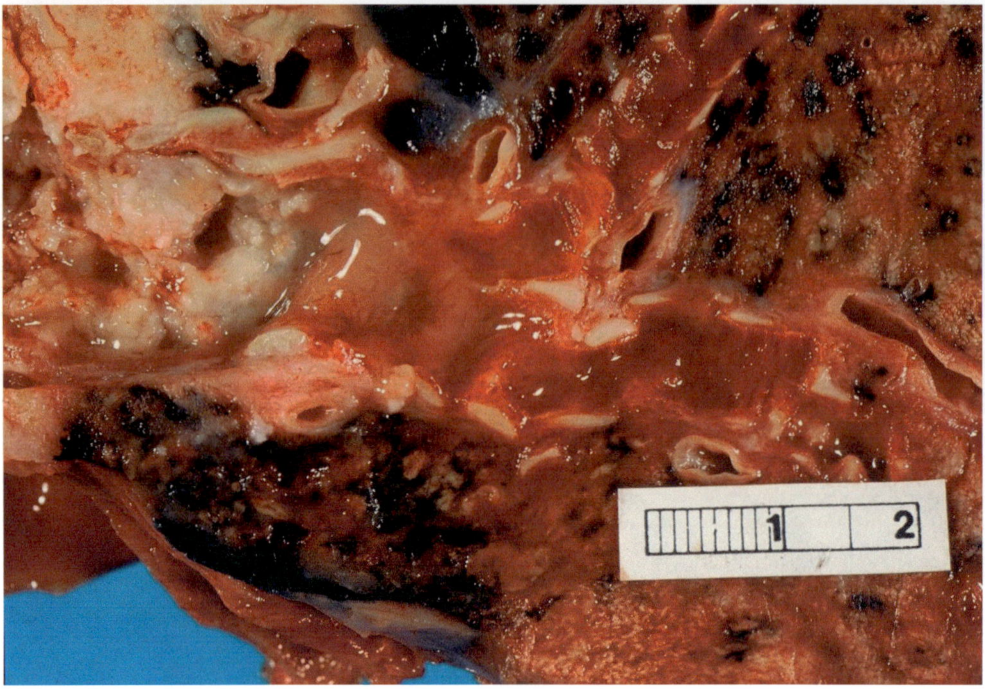

The biopsy taken at bronchoscopy is sent to the histopathology laboratory for microscopic examination in order to obtain a precise histological diagnosis, as well as for immunohistochemistry and genomic testing.

Figure X. Histopathology of a clear cell adenocarcinoma of the lung

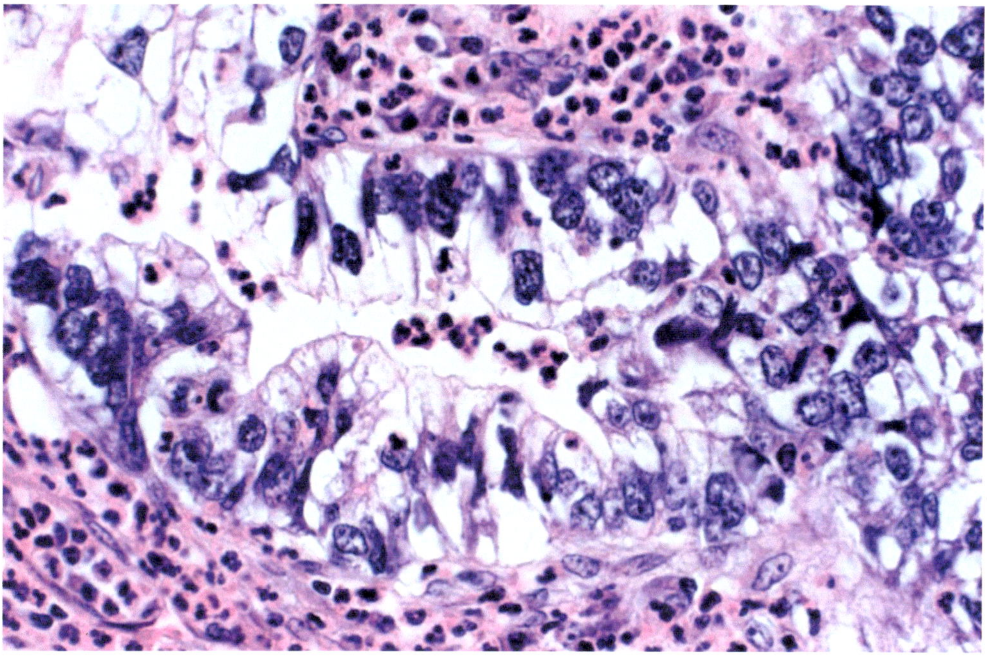

This image is by The Armed Forces Institute of Pathology (AFIP) - PEIR Digital Library (Pathology image database). Image# 407853. Public Domain, https://commons.wikimedia.org/w/index.php?curid=4356886; ommons.wikimedia.org/wiki/Category:Histopathology_of_adenocarcinomas_of_the_human_lung#/media/File:Clear_cell_adeno carcinoma_of_the_lung.jpg. This work is in the public domain in the United States because it is a work prepared by an officer or employee of the United States Government as part of that person's official duties under the terms of Title 17, Chapter 1, Section 105 of the US Code. No changes were made to this image.

Figure X. A lobectomy specimen showing a lobulated, somewhat glistening mass. Histopathology of this lesion showed it to be an adenocarcinoma of the lung.

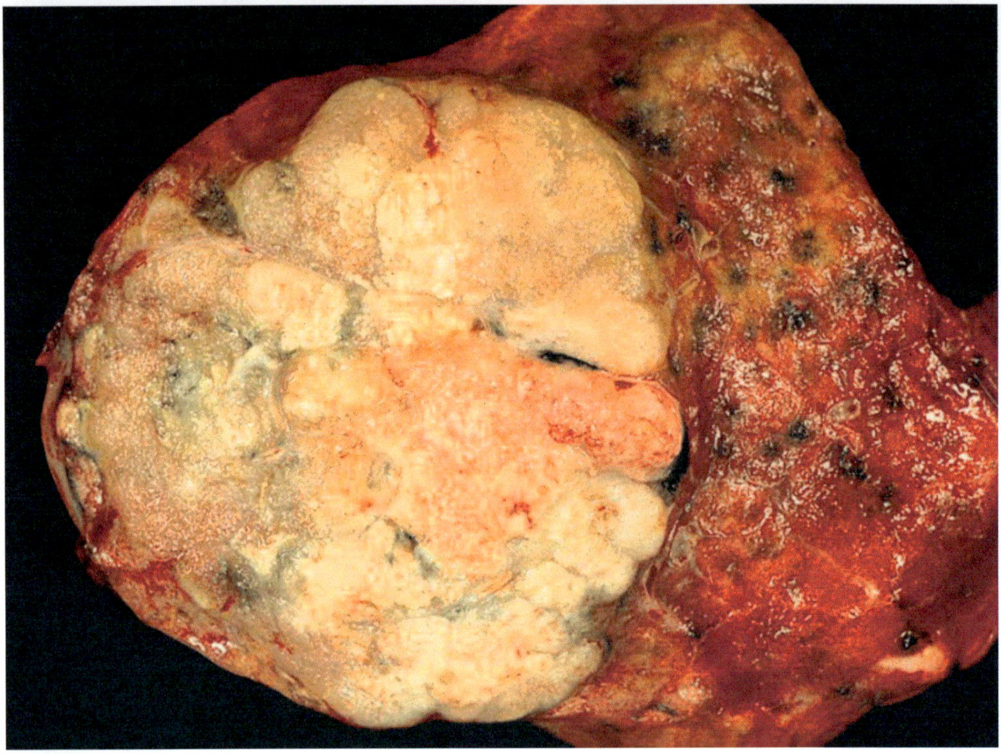

Staging of NSCLC

The TNM (tumor, node, metastasis) staging system is used for lung cancer:

- T Tumor

T1a: Primary tumor is ≤1 cm in greatest dimension.

T1b: Primary tumor is >1 but ≤2 cm in greatest dimension.

T1c: Primary tumor is >2 but ≤3 cm in greatest dimension.

T2a: Primary tumor is >3 and ≤5 cm in greatest dimension.

T2b: Primary tumor is >5 and ≤7 cm in greatest dimension.

T3size: Primary tumor is >7 cm in greatest dimension;

T3inv: Primary tumor invades the chest wall, diaphragm, phrenic nerve, mediastinal pleura, or pericardium;

T3centr: Primary tumor is <2 cm to the carina or there is atelectasis of the entire lung;

T3satell: Primary tumor is associated with separate tumor nodule(s) in same pulmonary lobe;

T4inv: Tumor invading the heart, great vessels, trachea, recurrent laryngeal nerve, esophagus, or spine;

T4ipsi: Tumor of any size with additional tumor nodule(s) in a different ipsilateral lobe;

- N Lymph node

N1 : Nodal metastasis in ipsilateral pulmonary or hilar lymph nodes;

N2 : Nodal metastasis in ipsilateral mediastinal/subcarinal lymph nodes;

- M Metastases other than to ipsilateral intrathoracic lymph nodes

M0, none present

M1: present

Treatment

Treatment of NSCLC depends upon the stage of the disease. Surgery is used for early disease which is localized in nature. More advanced disease is usually treated with cytotoxic chemotherapy and radiation. Recently, checkpoint inhibiors have shown significant efficacy: these drugs block the tumor-induced suppression of the patient's immune system and thus enable it to help in the treatment approach. Several small inhibitory molecules (tyrosine kinase inhibitors) are used if certain mutations are detected in the tumor: Patients with non-squamous NSCLC should have their tumor tested for the presence of a driver mutation, such as mutated epidermal growth factor receptor (*EGFR*), the anaplastic lymphoma kinase (*ALK*) fusion oncogene, and other targetable mutations. Also, a number of additional genetic markers are known to be mutated within NSCLC and may impact treatment in the future, including BRAF, HER2/neu, and KRAS. For advanced NSCLC, a combined chemotherapy treatment approach that includes cetuximab, an antibody that targets the EGFR signalling pathway, is more effective.

EGFR mutations

Roughly 10–35% of people who have NSCLC will have drug-sensitizing mutations of the EGFR. These people have been shown to be sensitive to certain medications that block the EGFR protein known as tyrosine kinase inhibitors specifically, **erlotinib, gefitinib, afatinib, or osimertinib**. **Lazertinib** was approved for medical use in the United States in August 2024. For patients with advanced NSCLC with EGFR exon 19 deletions or exon 21 L858R, **osimertinib** as the frontline treatment is generally preferred rather than other systemic treatment options. The combination of amivantamab (a monoclonal antibody that inhibits the EGFR) plus lazertinib has shown better progression-free survival benefit than osimertinib. However, the effect on overall survival is unknown, but this combination is recognized as an acceptable alternative to osimertinib. Lazertinib is currently only approved by the FDA for NSCLC when it is used in combination with the bispecific monoclonal antibody amivantamab.

ALK gene rearrangements

Up to 7% of NSCLC patients have EML4-ALK translocations or mutations in the ROS1 gene. These patients may benefit from ALK inhibitors, which are now approved for this subset of patients. **Crizotinib**, which gained FDA approval in August 2011, is an inhibitor of several kinases, specifically ALK, ROS1, and MET. Crizotinib has been shown in clinical studies to have response rates around 60% in patients shown to have ALK-positive disease. For those with newly diagnosed, ALK-positive NSCLC, a next-generation ALK inhibitor as first-line treatment rather than crizotinib is now preferred. In choosing between second-generation inhibitors, **alectinib** is preferred, given the benefit of longer-term follow-up of clinical trials with this agent compared with others. However, direct comparisons between second-generation inhibitors have not been performed, and thus **brigatinib** or **lorlatinib** are other acceptable front-line options.

Several studies have also shown that ALK mutations and EGFR activating mutations are typically mutually exclusive. Thus, it is not recommended that patients who fail crizotinib be switched to an EGFR-targeted drug.

The rest of this book will focus on the FDA approvals given for osimertinib, lazertinib, alectinib, brigatinib and lorlatinib using the FDA Highlights of Prescribing document and the FDA Full Prescribing Information on each drug.

7. Small inhibitory molecules (tyrosine kinase inhibitors) in the treatment of non-small cell lung cancer

7.1. Drug-sensitizing mutations of the epidermal growth factor receptor (EGFR)

(i) Osimertinib (TAGRISSO)

HIGHLIGHTS OF PRESCRIBING

1. INDICATIONS AND USAGE

TAGRISSO is a kinase inhibitor indicated for:

- adjuvant therapy after tumor resection in adult patients with non-small cell lung cancer (NSCLC) whose tumors have epidermal growth factor receptor (EGFR) exon 19 deletions or exon 21 L858R mutations, as detected by an FDA-approved test

- the first-line treatment of adult patients with metastatic NSCLC whose tumors have EGFR exon 19 deletions or exon 21 L858R mutations, as detected by an FDA-approved test.

- in combination with pemetrexed and platinum-based chemotherapy, the first-line treatment of adult patients with locally advanced or metastatic NSCLC whose tumors have EGFR exon 19 deletions or exon 21 L858R mutations, as detected by an FDA-approved test.

• the treatment of adult patients with metastatic EGFR T790M mutation positive NSCLC, as detected by an FDA-approved test, whose disease has progressed on or after EGFR TKI therapy.

12.1 MECHANISM OF ACTION

Osimertinib is a kinase inhibitor of the epidermal growth factor receptor (EGFR), which binds irreversibly to certain mutant forms of EGFR (T790M, L858R, and exon 19 deletion) at approximately 9 fold lower concentrations than wild-type. Two pharmacologically-active metabolites (AZ7550 and AZ5104 circulating at approximately 10% of the parent) with similar inhibitory profiles to osimertinib have been identified in the plasma after oral administration of osimertinib. AZ7550 showed a similar potency to osimertinib, while AZ5104 showed greater potency against exon 19 deletion and T790M mutants (approximately 8-fold) and wild-type (approximately 15-fold) EGFR. In vitro, osimertinib also inhibited the activity of HER2, HER3, HER4, ACK1, and BLK at clinically relevant concentrations. In cultured cells and animal tumor implantation models, osimertinib exhibited anti-tumor activity against NSCLC lines harboring EGFR-mutations (T790M/L858R, L858R, T790M/exon 19 deletion, and exon 19 deletion) and, to a lesser extent, wild-type EGFR amplifications. Osimertinib distributed to the brain in 14 multiple animal species (monkey, rat, and mouse) with brain to plasma AUC ratios of approximately 2 following oral dosing. These data are consistent with observations of tumor regression and increased survival in osimertinib versus control-treated animals in a pre-clinical mutant-EGFR intracranial mouse metastasis xenograft model (PC9; exon 19 deletion).

DOSAGE AND ADMINISTRATION

Adjuvant treatment of early stage NSCLC

80 mg orally once daily, with or without food, until disease recurrence, or unacceptable toxicity, or for up to 3 years.

Metastatic NSCLC

80 mg orally once daily, with or without food, until disease progression or unacceptable toxicity.

DOSAGE FORMS AND STRENGTHS

Tablets: 80 mg and 40 mg.

80 mg tablets: beige, oval and biconvex tablet marked with “AZ 80” on one side and plain on the reverse. 40 mg tablets: beige, round and biconvex tablet marked with “AZ 40” on one side and plain on the reverse.

CONTRAINDICATIONS

None

WARNINGS AND PRECAUTIONS

- Interstitial lung disease (ILD)/pneumonitis: occurred in 3.7% of patients. Permanently discontinue TAGRISSO in patients diagnosed with ILD/Pneumonitis.

((Interstitial lung disease, or diffuse parenchymal lung disease, is a group of respiratory diseases affecting the interstitium (the tissue) and space around the alveoli (air sacs) of the lungs. In interstitial lung disease, the tissue around the air sacs (alveoli) becomes scarred and thickened. This makes it more difficult for oxygen to pass into the bloodstream. The disease presents with shortness of breath, nonproductive cough, fatigue, and weight loss, which tend to develop slowly, over several months).

(Figure X. A diagram of the alveoli).

(This image is by By LadyofHats - Own work using:Image:Respiratory system complete.svg) (duplicate of Image:Respiratory system complete en.svg), Public Domain, https://commons.wikimedia.org/w/index.php?curid=3222341; en.wikipedia.org/wiki/Interstitial_lung_disease#/media/File:Alveolus_diagram.svg. This work has been released into the public domain by its author, LadyofHats. No changes were made to this image).

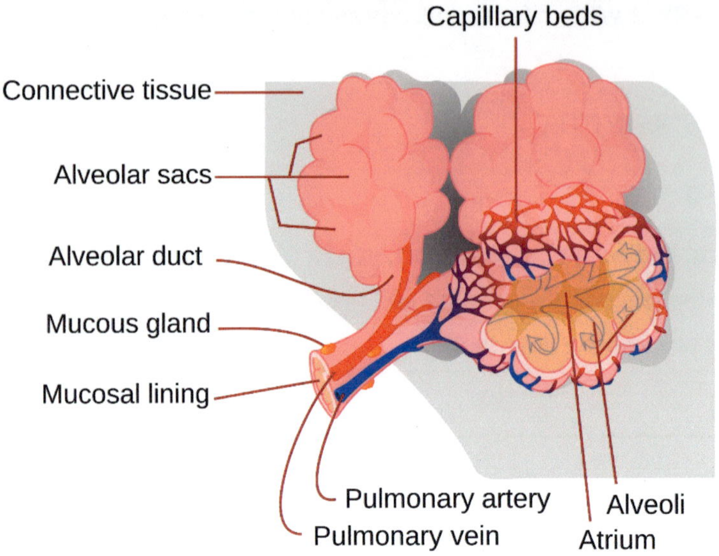

(Figure X. A chest x-ray showing interstitial markings. In this case the interstitial pneumonitis was due to Pneumocystis jiroveci infection).

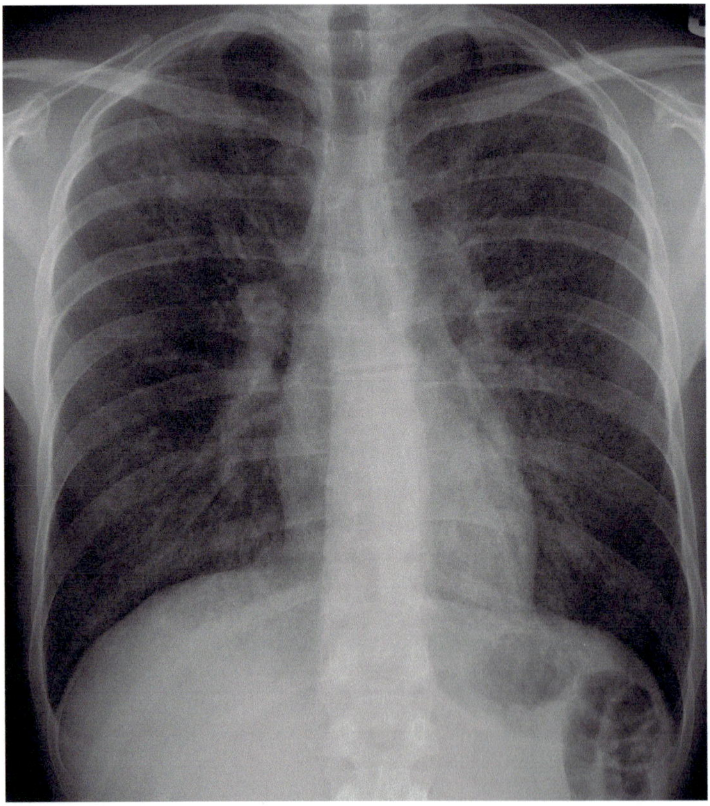

(This image is by Samir Public Domain, https://commons.wikimedia.org/w/index.php?curid=85067168; en.wikipedia.org/wiki/Interstitial_lung_disease#/media/File:PCP_CAP_CXR.JPG. The copyright holder of this work has released this work into the public domain. No changes were made to this image).

QTc interval prolongation: monitor electrocardiograms and electrolytes in patients who have a history or predisposition for QTc prolongation, or those who are taking medications that are known to prolong the QTc interval. Withhold then restart at a reduced dose or permanently discontinue TAGRISSO.

(Figure X. Schematic diagram of sinus rhythm for a human heart as seen on an echocardiogram: the QT interval is shown).

(This image is by Agateller (Anthony Atkielski), converted to svg by atom. - SinusRhythmLabels.png, Public Domain, https://commons.wikimedia.org/w/index.php?curid=1560893; en.wikipedia.org/wiki/Electrocardiography#/media/File:SinusRhythmLabels.svg. the copyright holder of this work, release this work into the public domain. No changes were made to this image).

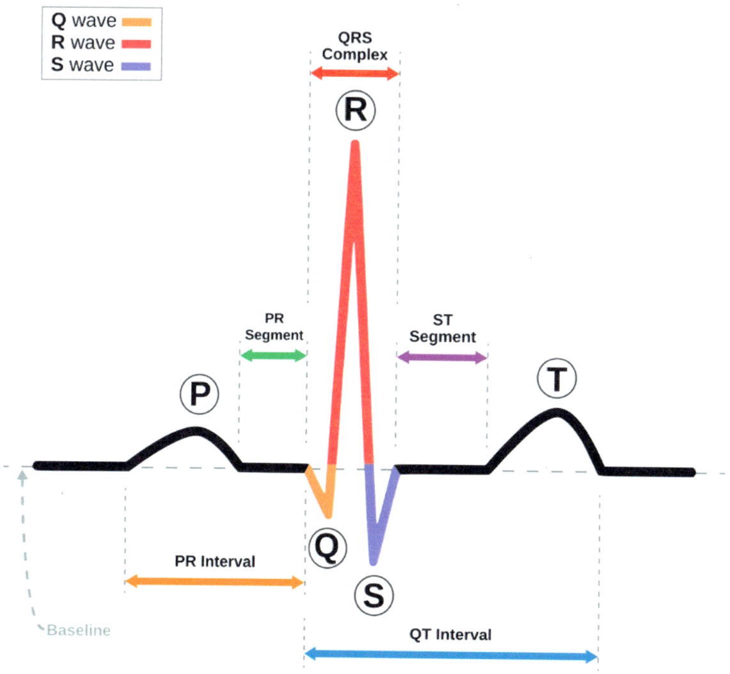

(The QTc is the QT interval corrected for heart rate according to the formulae seen in Figure X.

Figure X. QT interval corrected for heart rate)

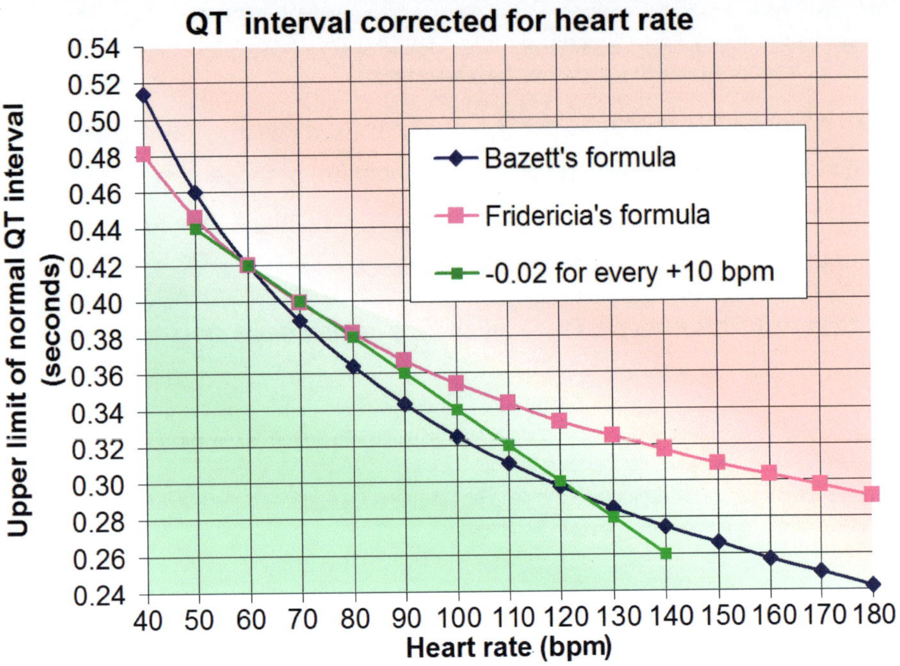

(This image is by Mikael Häggström. https://commons.wikimedia.org/w/index.php?curid=9822028; en.wikipedia.org/wiki/QT_interval#/media/File:QT_interval_corrected_for_heart_rate.png. The copyright holder of this work has released this work into the public domain. No changes were made to this image).

- Cardiomyopathy: occurred in 3% of patients. Conduct cardiac monitoring, including left ventricular ejection fraction (LVEF) assessment in patients with cardiac risk factors.

(Figure X. Gross pathology of idiopathic cardiomyopathy. Opened left ventricle of heart shows a thickened, dilated left ventricle with subendocardial fibrosis manifested as increased whiteness of endocardium. Autopsy).

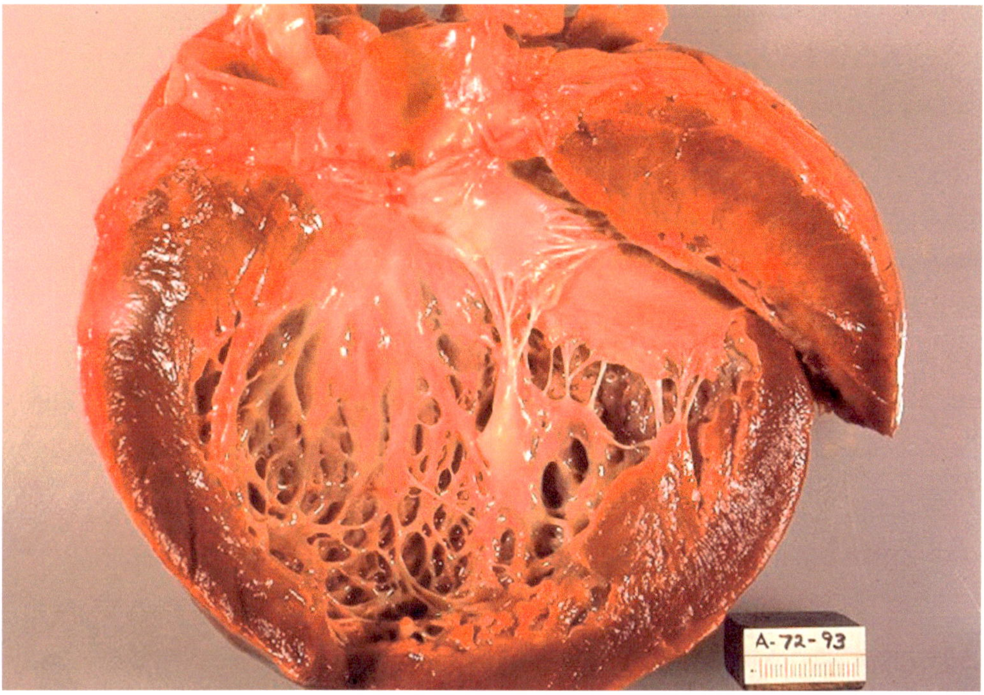

(This image is by CDC/Dr. Edwin P. Ewing, Jr. - http://phil.cdc.gov/PHIL_Images/02051999/00018/20G0018_lores.jpg, Public Domain, https://commons.wikimedia.org/w/index.php?curid=825652; en.wikipedia.org/wiki/Cardiomyopathy#/media/File:Idiopathic_cardiomyopathy,_gross_pathology_20G0018_lores.jpg. This image is a work of the Centers for Disease Control and Prevention, part of the United States Department of Health and Human Services, taken or made as part of an employee's official duties. As a work of the U.S. federal government, the image is in the public domain. No changes were made to this image).

- Keratitis: promptly refer patients with signs and symptoms of keratitis to an ophthalmologist for evaluation.

(Keratitis is a condition in which the becomes inflamed. The condition is often marked by moderate to intense pain and usually involves any of the following symptoms: pain, impaired eyesight, photophobia (light sensitivity), red eye and a 'gritty' sensation. Diagnosis of infectious keratitis is usually made clinically based on the signs and symptoms as well as eye examination).

- Erythema multiforme and Stevens-Johnson syndrome: withhold TAGRISSO if erythema multiforme major or Stevens-Johnson syndrome is suspected and permanently discontinue if confirmed.

(The rash of Erythema multiforme involves erythematous patches evolving into target lesions (which blanche on pressure), typically on both hands), but it can spread to the rest of the skin and can also involve the oral mucous membrane).

(Stevens–Johnson syndrome (SJS) is a type of severe skin reaction. It overlaps with toxic epidermal necrolysis (TEN). They are considered febrile mucocutaneous drug reactions and probably part of the same spectrum of disease, with SJS being less severe. Erythema multiforme is generally considered a separate condition. Early symptoms of SJS include fever and flu-like symptoms. A few days later, the skin begins to blister and peel, forming painful raw areas. Mucous membranes, such as the mouth, are also typically involved. Complications include dehydration, sepsis, pneumonia and multiple organ failure).

- Cutaneous vasculitis: withhold TAGRISSO if cutaneous vasculitis is suspected, evaluate for systemic involvement, and consider dermatology consultation. If no other etiology can be identified, consider permanent discontinuation based on severity.

(Cutaneous small-vessel vasculitis is inflammation of small blood vessels, usually accompanied by small lumps beneath the skin. The condition is also known as hypersensitivity vasculitis, cutaneous leukocytoclastic vasculitis, hypersensitivity angiitis, cutaneous leukocytoclastic angiitis, cutaneous necrotizing vasculitis and cutaneous necrotizing venulitis. It is the most common form of vasculitis seen in clinical practice, usually caused by inflammation of post-capillary venules in the dermis). "Leukocytoclastic" (literally meaning 'leukocyte-destroying') refers to the damage caused by nuclear debris from infiltrating neutrophils in and around the vessels. Initially red to pink, flat spots (macules) and raised bumps (papules) may be seen on the skin. Once fully developed, the classic appearance is "non-blanching, palpable purpura". This appears as deep red to purple spots that feel raised to the touch. When gently pressed, the color does not fade to a lighter color ("non-blanching"). Small fluid-filled blisters (vesicles), pus-filled bumps resembling a pimple (pustules), or shallow ulcers may also develop but are less common. The location of skin lesions varies but are most commonly found symmetrically below the waist, primarily on the buttocks and legs. Other distributions include localized areas on the upper body or

over several areas of the body. With treatment, the lesions typically resolve in weeks to months and leave behind flat spots that are darker than the surrounding skin (postinflammatory hyperpigmentation).

- Embryo-Fetal Toxicity: TAGRISSO can cause fetal harm. Advise females of potential risk to the fetus and to use effective contraception during treatment with TAGRISSO and for 6 weeks after final dose. Advise males to use effective contraception for 4 months, after the last dose of TAGRISSO.

ADVERSE REACTIONS

- Most common (>20%) adverse reactions, including laboratory abnormalities were leukopenia, lymphopenia, thrombocytopenia, diarrhea, anemia, rash, musculoskeletal pain, nail toxicity, neutropenia, dry skin, stomatitis, fatigue, and cough.

To report SUSPECTED ADVERSE REACTIONS, contact AstraZeneca at 1-800-236-9933 or www.TAGRISSO.com or FDA at 1-800-FDA-1088 or www.fda.gov/medwatch.

DRUG INTERACTIONS

Strong CYP3A inducers: avoid if possible. If not possible, increase TAGRISSO to 160 mg daily in patients receiving a strong CYP3A4 inducer.

(Strong CYP3A4 inducers include

Armodafinil

Barbiturates

Capsaicin

Carbamazepine

Efavirenz

Enzalutamide

Glucocorticoids

Modafinil

Nevirapine

Oxcarbazepine

Phenytoin

Pioglitazone

Quercetin

Rifabutin

Rifampicin

Rifapentine

St. John's wort

Topiramate

Troglitazone

USE IN SPECIFIC POPULATIONS

Lactation: do not breastfeed

4. CONTRAINDICATIONS
5. None.

1 4. CLINICAL STUDIES

14.1 Adjuvant treatment of early-stage EGFR mutation-positive non-small cell lung cancer

The efficacy of TAGRISSO was demonstrated in a randomized, double-blind, placebo controlled trial (ADAURA [NCT02511106]) for the adjuvant treatment of patients with EGFR exon 19 deletions or exon 21 L858R mutation-positive NSCLC who had complete tumor resection, with or without prior adjuvant chemotherapy. Eligible patients with resectable tumors (stage IB – IIIA according to American Joint Commission on Cancer [AJCC] 7th edition) were required to have predominantly non-squamous histology and EGFR exon 19 deletions or exon 21 L858R mutations identified prospectively from tumor tissue in a central laboratory by the cobas®

EGFR Mutation Test. Patients with clinically significant uncontrolled cardiac disease, prior history of ILD/pneumonitis, or who received treatment with any EGFR kinase inhibitor were not eligible for the study. Patients were randomized (1:1) to receive TAGRISSO 80 mg orally once daily or placebo following recovery from surgery and standard adjuvant chemotherapy if given. Patients who did not receive adjuvant chemotherapy were randomized within 10 weeks and patients who received adjuvant chemotherapy were randomized within 26 weeks following surgery. Randomization was stratified by mutation type (exon 19 deletions or exon 21 L858R mutations), race (Asian or non-Asian) and pTNM staging (IB or II or IIIA) according to AJCC 7th edition. Treatment was given for 3 years or until disease recurrence, or unacceptable toxicity. The major efficacy outcome measure was disease-free survival (DFS, defined as reduction in the risk of disease recurrence or death) in patients with stage II – IIIA NSCLC determined by investigator assessment. Additional efficacy outcome measures included DFS in the overall population (patients with stage IB – IIIA NSCLC), and overall survival (OS) in patients with stage II – IIIA NSCLC and in the overall population. A total of 682 patients were randomized to TAGRISSO (n=339) or placebo (n=343). The median age was 63 years (range 30-86 years); 70% were female; 64% were Asian and 72% were never TAGRISSO® (osimertinib) tablets, for oral use smokers. Baseline World Health Organization (WHO) performance status was 0 (64%) or 1 (36%); 31% had stage IB, 35% II, and 34% IIIA. With regard to EGFR mutation status, 55% were exon 19 deletions and 45% were exon 21 L858R mutations. The majority (60%) of patients received adjuvant chemotherapy prior to randomization (27% IB; 70% II, 79% IIIA). ADAURA demonstrated a statistically significant difference in DFS for patients treated with TAGRISSO compared to patients treated with placebo. The final analysis of OS demonstrated a statistically significant improvement in OS for patients treated with TAGRISSO compared to patients treated with placebo. Median OS was not reached in either arm. In the overall population (IB-IIIA), the median follow-up time was 61.5 months in both treatment arms.

14.2. Previously untreated EGFR mutation-positive metastatic NSCLC

The efficacy of TAGRISSO was demonstrated in a randomized, multicenter, double-blind, active controlled trial (FLAURA [NCT02296125]) in patients with EGFR exon 19 deletions or exon 21 L858R mutation-positive, metastatic NSCLC, who had not received previous systemic treatment for metastatic disease. Patients were required to have measurable disease per RECIST v1.1, a WHO performance status of 0-1, and EGFR exon 19 deletions or exon 21 L858R mutation in tumor prospectively identified by the cobas® EGFR Mutation Test in a central laboratory or by an investigational assay at a CLIA-certified or accredited laboratory. Patients with CNS metastases not requiring steroids and with stable neurologic status for at least two weeks after completion of definitive surgery or radiotherapy were eligible. Patients were assessed at the investigator's discretion for CNS metastases if they had a history of, or suspected, CNS metastases at study entry. Patients were randomized (1:1) to receive TAGRISSO 80 mg orally once daily or to receive gefitinib 250 mg orally once daily or erlotinib 150 mg orally once daily until disease progression or unacceptable toxicity. Randomization was stratified by EGFR mutation type (exon 19 deletions or exon 21 L858R mutation) and ethnicity (Asian or non-Asian). Patients randomized to the control arm were offered TAGRISSO at the time of disease progression if tumor samples tested positive for the EGFR T790M mutation. The major efficacy outcome measure was progression-free survival (PFS), as assessed by investigator. Additional efficacy outcome measures included OS and overall response rate (ORR). A total of 556 patients were randomized to TAGRISSO (n=279) or to control (gefitinib n=183; erlotinib n=94). The median age was 64 years (range 26-93 years); 54% were < 65 years of age; 63% were female; 62% were Asian and 64% were never smokers. Baseline WHO performance status was 0 (41%) or 1 (59%); 5% had Stage IIIb and 95% had Stage IV; and 7% received prior systemic cytotoxic chemotherapy as neoadjuvant or adjuvant therapy. With regard to EGFR tumor testing, 63% were exon 19 deletions and 37% were exon 21 L858R; 5 patients (<1%) also had a concomitant de novo T790M mutation. EGFR mutation status was confirmed centrally using the cobas® EGFR Mutation Test in 90% of patients. At the time of the final data cut-off, of those randomized to TAGRISSO and to investigator's choice erlotinib or gefitinib arm, 133 (48%) and 180 (65%) patients had received at least one subsequent treatment, respectively. Out of the 180 patients randomized to erlotinib or gefitinib who received subsequent treatment, 85 (47%) patients received TAGRISSO as first subsequent therapy. FLAURA demonstrated a statistically significant improvement in PFS for patients randomized to TAGRISSO as compared to erlotinib or gefitinib. The final analysis of overall survival demonstrated a statistically significant improvement in overall survival in patients randomized to TAGRISSO compared to erlotinib or gefitinib.

(ii) **LAZERTINIB**

LAZCLUZE™ (lazertinib) tablets, for oral use. Initial U.S. Approval: 2024

INDICATIONS AND USAGE

LAZCLUZE is a kinase inhibitor indicated in combination with amivantamab for the first-line treatment of adult patients with locally advanced or metastatic non-small cell lung cancer (NSCLC) with epidermal growth factor receptor (EGFR) exon 19 deletions or exon 21 L858R substitution mutations, as detected by an FDA-approved test.

(Amivantamab is a bispecific epidermal growth factor (EGF) receptor-directed and mesenchymal–epithelial transition (MET) receptor-directed antibody).

(Figure X. Cartoon diagram of the epidermal growth factor receptor (EGFR) (rainbow colored, N-terminus = blue, C-terminus = red) complexed its ligand epidermal growth factor (magenta) based on the PDB: 1NQL crystallographic coordinates).

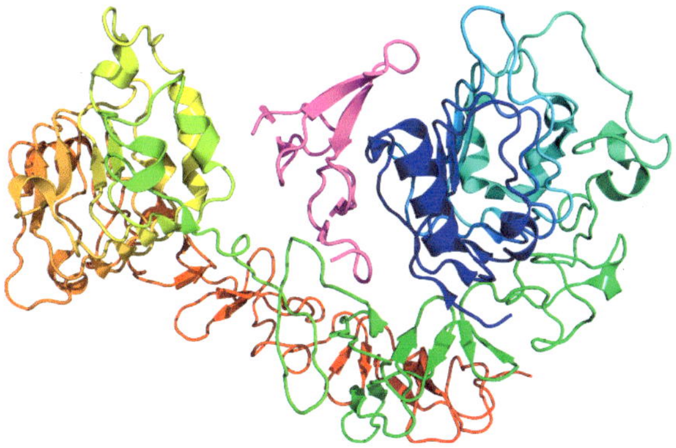

Mechanism of Action

Lazertinib is a kinase inhibitor of epidermal growth factor receptor (EGFR) that inhibits EGFR exon 19 deletions and exon 21 L858R substitution mutations at lower concentrations than wild type EGFR. In human NSCLC cells and mouse xenograft models of EGFR exon 19 deletions or EGFR L858R substitution mutations, lazertinib demonstrated anti-tumor activity. Treatment with lazertinib in combination with amivantamab increased in vivo anti-tumor activity compared to either agent alone in a mouse xenograft model of human NSCLC with an EGFR L858R mutation

DOSAGE AND ADMINISTRATION

• The recommended dosage of LAZCLUZE is 240 mg orally once daily with or without food, given in combination with amivantamab.

• Continue treatment until disease progression or unacceptable toxicity.

• Administer LAZCLUZE any time prior to amivantamab when given on the same day.

• Refer to the amivantamab prescribing information for recommended amivantamab dosing information.

• Administer anticoagulant prophylaxis to prevent venous thromboembolic events for the first four months of treatment.

DOSAGE FORMS AND STRENGTHS

Tablets:80 mg and 240 mg.

CONTRAINDICATIONS

None.

WARNINGS AND PRECAUTIONS

• Venous Thromboembolic Events (VTE): prophylactic anticoagulation is recommended for the first four months of treatment. Monitor for signs and symptoms of VTE and treat as medically appropriate. Withhold LAZCLUZE and amivantamab based on severity. Once anticoagulant treatment has been initiated, resume LAZCLUZE and amivantamab at the same dose at the discretion of the healthcare provider. Permanently discontinue amivantamab and continue LAZCLUZE for recurrent VTE despite therapeutic anticoagulation.

(Venous thromboembolism includes deep vein thrombosis only (DVT) , DVT with pulmonary embolism (PE), and PE only.

Figure X. A chest CT scan showing a pulmonary embolism (white arrow) that has been long-standing and has caused a lung infarction (black arrow) seen as a reverse halo sign).

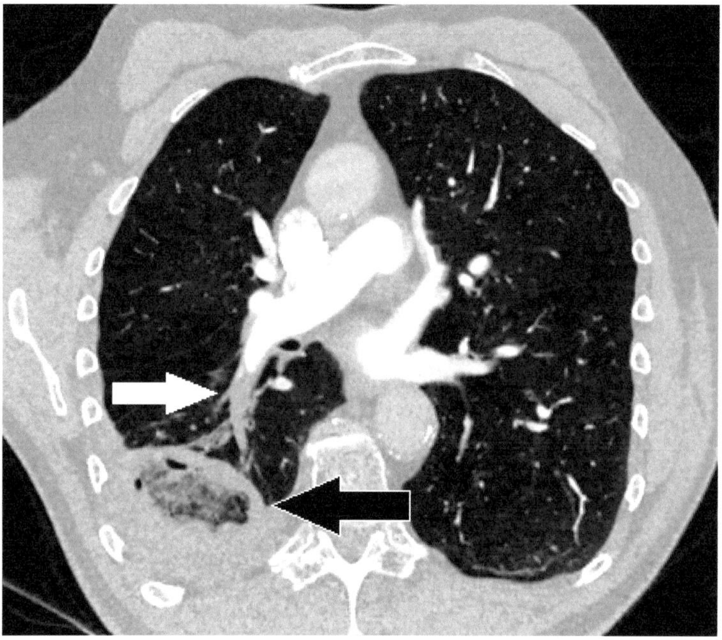

(This image is by Mikael Häggström, M.D. Author info- Reusing images- Conflicts of interest:NoneMikael Häggström, M.D.Consent note: Written informed consent was obtained from the individual, including online publication. - Own work, CC0, https://commons.wikimedia.org/w/index.php?curid=76743775; https://en.wikipedia.org/wiki/Pulmonary_embolism#/media/File:CT_of_lung_infarction_with_reverse_halo_sign,_annotated.png. This file is made available under the Creative Commons CC0 1.0 Universal Public Domain Dedication. No changes were made to this image).

- Interstitial Lung Disease (ILD)/Pneumonitis

Monitor for new or worsening symptoms indicative of ILD/pneumonitis. Withhold LAZCLUZE and amivantamab in patients with suspected ILD/pneumonitis and permanently discontinue if ILD/pneumonitis is confirmed.

- Dermatologic adverse reactions

May cause severe rash including acneiform dermatitis. Administer alcohol-free emollient cream and encourage patients to limit sun exposure during and for 2 months after treatment to reduce the risk of dermatologic reactions. Withhold, reduce the dose or permanently discontinue LAZCLUZE and amivantamab based on severity.

Figure X. Teenager with acne

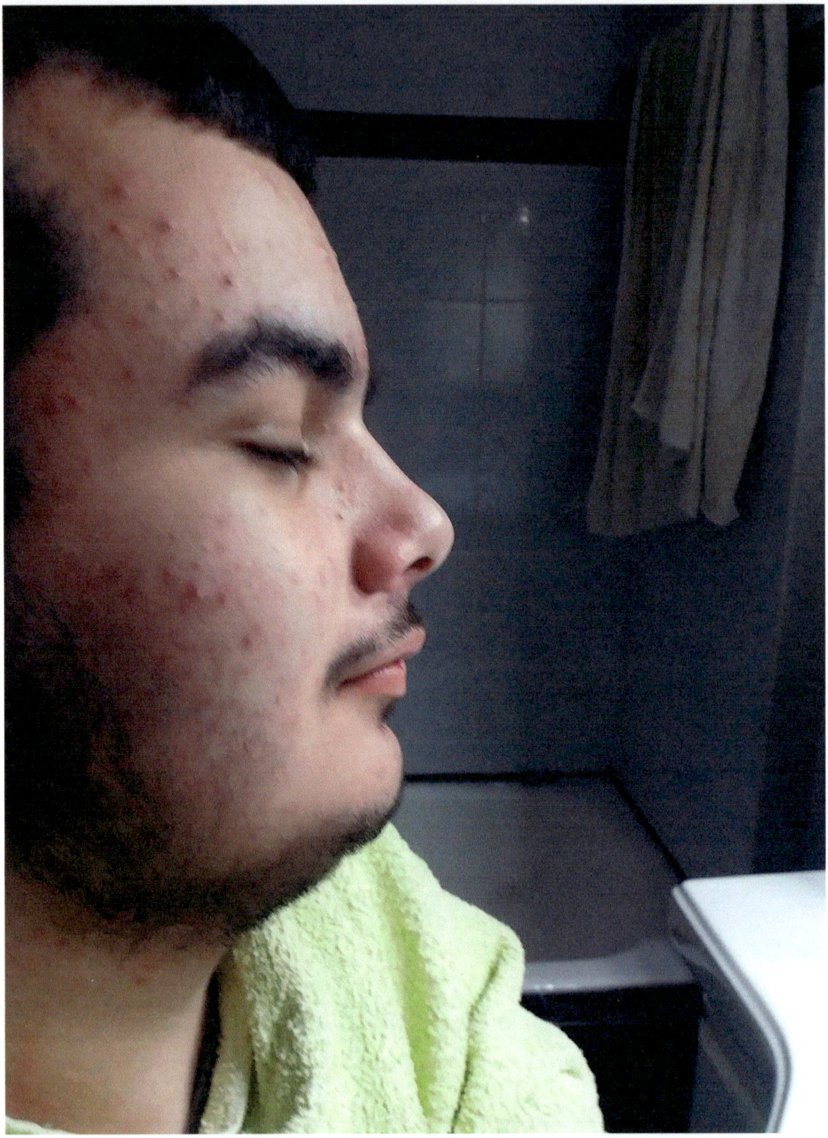

(This image is by NikosLikomitros - Own work, CC0, https://commons.wikimedia.org/w/index.php?curid=127724206; https://en.wikipedia.org/wiki/Acne#/media/File:Teenager_with_acne.jpg. The copyright holder of this work has made it available under the Creative Commons CC0 1.0 Universal Public Domain Dedication. No changes were made to this image).

• Ocular adverse reactions

Promptly refer patients with new or worsening signs and symptoms of ocular adverse reactions, including keratitis, to an ophthalmologist for evaluation. Withhold, reduce the dose, or permanently discontinue amivantamab and continue LAZCLUZE based on severity.

• Embryo-Fetal Toxicity

Can cause fetal harm. Advise patients of reproductive potential of the potential risk to a fetus and to use effective contraception.

ADVERSE REACTIONS

LAZCLUZE in combination with amivantamab

• The most common adverse reactions (≥ 20%) were rash, nail toxicity, infusion-related reaction (amivantamab), musculoskeletal pain, edema, stomatitis, VTE, paresthesia, fatigue, diarrhea, constipation, COVID-19, hemorrhage, dry skin, decreased appetite, pruritus, nausea, and ocular toxicity.

• The most common Grade 3 or 4 laboratory abnormalities (≥ 2%) were decreased albumin, decreased sodium, increased ALT, decreased potassium, decreased hemoglobin, increased AST, increased GGT, and increased magnesium. To report SUSPECTED ADVERSE REACTIONS, contact Janssen Biotech, Inc. at 1-800-526-7736 or FDA at 1-800-FDA-1088 or www.fda.gov/medwatch.

DRUG INTERACTIONS

Strong and moderate CYP3A4 inducers: avoid concomitant use.

USE IN SPECIFIC POPULATIONS

Pregnancy

Lactation: advise not to breastfeed.

CLINICAL STUDIES

The efficacy of LAZCLUZE, in combination with amivantamab, was evaluated in MARIPOSA [NCT04487080], a randomized, active-controlled, multicenter trial. Eligible patients were required to have untreated locally advanced or metastatic

NSCLC with either exon 19 deletions or exon 21 L858R substitution EGFR mutations identified by local testing, not amenable to curative therapy. Patients with asymptomatic or previously treated and stable intracranial metastases were eligible to enroll. Patients were randomized (2:2:1) to receive LAZCLUZE in combination with amivantamab (N=429), osimertinib monotherapy (N=429), or LAZCLUZE monotherapy (an unapproved regimen for NSCLC) until disease progression or unacceptable toxicity. The evaluation of efficacy for the treatment of untreated metastatic NSCLC relied upon comparison between:

• LAZCLUZE administered at 240 mg orally once daily in combination with amivantamab administered intravenously at 1050 mg (for patients < 80 kg) or 1400 mg (for patients ≥ 80 kg) once weekly for 4 weeks, then every 2 weeks thereafter starting at week 5.

• Osimertinib administered at a dose of 80 mg orally once daily. Randomization was stratified by EGFR mutation type (exon 19 deletion or exon 21 L858R substitution mutation), Asian race (yes or no), and history of brain metastasis (yes or no). Tumor assessments were performed every 8 weeks for 30 months, and then every 12 weeks until disease progression.

The major efficacy outcome measure was progression-free survival (PFS) as assessed by blinded independent central review (BICR). Additional efficacy outcome measures included overall survival (OS), overall response rate (ORR) and duration of response (DOR). A total of 858 patients were randomized between the two study arms, 429 to the LAZCLUZE in combination with amivantamab arm and 429 to the osimertinib arm. The median age was 63 (range: 25–88) years; 61% were female; 58% were Asian, and 38% were White, 1.6% were American Indian or Alaska Native, 0.8% were Black or African American, 0.2% were Native Hawaiian or other Pacific Islander, 0.6% were unknown race or multiple races; and 12% were Hispanic or Latino. Eastern Cooperative Oncology Group (ECOG) performance status was 0 (34%) or 1 (66%); 69% never smoked; 41% had prior brain metastases; and 89% had Stage IV cancer at initial diagnosis. Sixty percent of patients had tumors harboring exon 19 deletions and the remaining 40% had exon 21 L858R substitution mutations. Among the 858 patients with EGFR exon 19 deletion or L858R substitution mutations that were randomized between the amivantamab plus

LAZCLUZE arm versus the osimertinib arm, available tissue samples from 544 (63%) patients had evaluable results when tested retrospectively using the cobas EGFR Mutation Test v2. Of the 544 patients with evaluable results, 527 (97%) patients were positive for EGFR exon 19 deletion or L858R substitution mutations, while 17 (3%) patients were negative. Available plasma samples from patients were retrospectively tested using an FDA approved test to confirm the biomarker status.

The trial demonstrated a statistically significant improvement in PFS by BICR assessment for LAZCLUZE in combination with amivantamab compared to osimertinib alone.

8.2. Drug-sensitizing mutations of the anaplastic lymphoma kinase gene

(i) Alectinib (ALECENZA)

INDICATIONS AND USAGE

ALECENSA is a kinase inhibitor indicated for:

• adjuvant treatment in adult patients following tumor resection of anaplastic lymphoma kinase (ALK)-positive non-small cell lung cancer (NSCLC) (tumors ≥ 4 cm or node positive) as detected by an FDA approved test.

• treatment of adult patients with ALK-positive metastatic NSCLC as detected by an FDA-approved test.

DOSAGE AND ADMINISTRATION

600 mg orally twice daily. Administer ALECENSA with food.

DOSAGE FORMS AND STRENGTHS

Capsules: 150 mg

CONTRAINDICATIONS

None.

WARNINGS AND PRECAUTIONS

• Hepatotoxicity: monitor liver laboratory tests every 2 weeks during the first 3 months of treatment, then once a month and as clinically indicated, with more frequent testing in patients who develop transaminase and bilirubin elevations. In case of severe ALT, AST, or bilirubin elevations, withhold, then reduce dose, or permanently discontinue ALECENSA.

• Interstitial Lung Disease (ILD)/Pneumonitis: immediately withhold ALECENSA in patients diagnosed with ILD/pneumonitis and permanently discontinue if no other potential causes of ILD/pneumonitis have been identified.

• Renal Impairment: withhold ALECENSA for severe renal impairment, then resume ALECENSA at reduced dose upon recovery or permanently discontinue

• Bradycardia: monitor heart rate and blood pressure regularly. If symptomatic, withhold ALECENSA then reduce dose, or permanently discontinue.

• Severe myalgia and creatine phosphokinase (CPK) elevation: assess CPK every 2 weeks during the first month of treatment and in patients reporting unexplained muscle pain, tenderness, or weakness. In case of severe CPK elevations, withhold, then resume or reduce dose.

• Hemolytic anemia: if hemolytic anemia is suspected, withhold ALECENSA. If hemolytic anemia is confirmed, consider resuming at a reduced dose upon resolution or permanently discontinue.

- Embryo-Fetal Toxicity: ALECENSA can cause fetal harm. Advise females of reproductive potential of the potential risk to a fetus and to use effective contraception.
- ADVERSE REACTIONS

The most common adverse reactions (incidence ≥20%) were hepatotoxicity, constipation, fatigue, myalgia, edema, rash and cough. To report SUSPECTED ADVERSE REACTIONS, contact Genentech at 1-888-835-2555 or FDA at 1-800-FDA-1088 or www.fda.gov/medwatch.

USE IN SPECIFIC POPULATIONS

Pregnancy

Lactation: Do not breastfeed.

CLINICAL STUDIES

14.1 Adjuvant treatment of resected ALK-positive NSCLC

The efficacy of ALECENSA for the adjuvant treatment of patients with ALK-positive NSCLC following complete tumor resection was evaluated in a global, randomized open-label clinical trial (ALINA: NCT03456076). Eligible patients were required to have resectable ALK-positive NSCLC, Stage IB (tumors ≥ 4 cm) – IIIA per the Union for International Cancer Control/American Joint Committee on Cancer (UICC/AJCC) Staging System, 7th Edition. ALK rearrangements were identified by a locally performed FDA-approved ALK test or by a centrally performed VENTANA ALK (D5F3) CDx assay. Randomization was stratified by race (Asian vs. other races) and stage of disease (IB vs. II vs. IIIA).

Patients were randomized (1:1) to receive ALECENSA 600 mg orally twice daily or platinum-based chemotherapy following tumor resection. Treatment with ALECENSA continued for a total of 2 years, or until disease recurrence or unacceptable toxicity occurred. Platinum-based chemotherapy was administered intravenously for 4 cycles, with each cycle lasting 21 days, according to one of the following regimens:

- Cisplatin 75 mg/m2 on Day 1 plus vinorelbine 25 mg/m2 on Days 1 and 8

- Cisplatin 75 mg/m2 on Day 1 plus gemcitabine 1250 mg/m2 on Days 1 and 8

- Cisplatin 75 mg/m2 on Day 1 plus pemetrexed 500 mg/m2 on Day 1 In the event of intolerance to a cisplatin-based regimen, carboplatin was administered instead of cisplatin in the above combinations at a dose of AUC 5 mg/mL/min or 6 mg/mL/min.

The major efficacy outcome measures were disease-free survival (DFS) in patients with stage II-IIIA NSCLC and DFS in patients with stage IB-IIIA NSCLC (intent-to-treat [ITT] population) as assessed by investigator. DFS was defined as the time from date of randomization to the date of occurrence of any of the following: first documented recurrence of disease, new primary NSCLC, or death due to any cause, whichever occurred first. An additional efficacy outcome measure was overall survival (OS) in the ITT population. A total of 257 patients were randomized to ALECENSA (N=130) or to chemotherapy (N=127). The median age was 56 years (range: 26 to 87), 24% were ≥ 65 years old; 52% were female; 56% were Asian, 42% were White, 0.4% were Black or African American, 2.3% were race unknown; 0.4% were Hispanic or Latino; 60% were never smokers; 53% had an ECOG PS of 0; 10% of patients had Stage IB, 35% had Stage II and 55% had Stage IIIA disease.

ALINA demonstrated a statistically significant improvement in DFS for patients treated with ALECENSA compared to patients treated with chemotherapy. OS data were not mature at the time of DFS analysis with 2.3% of deaths reported in the ITT population.

(ii) **BRIGATINIB**

Initial U.S. Approval: 2017

RECENT MAJOR CHANGES

INDICATIONS AND USAGE

ALUNBRIG is a kinase inhibitor indicated for the treatment of adult patients with anaplastic lymphoma kinase (ALK)-positive metastatic non-small cell lung cancer (NSCLC) as detected by an FDA-approved test.

DOSAGE AND ADMINISTRATION

90 mg orally once daily for the first 7 days; then increase to 180 mg orally once daily. May be taken with or without food.

DOSAGE FORMS AND STRENGTHS

Tablets: 180 mg, 90 mg, or 30 mg.

CONTRAINDICATION

None.

WARNINGS AND PRECAUTIONS

• Interstitial Lung Disease (ILD)/Pneumonitis: monitor for new or worsening respiratory symptoms, particularly during the first week of treatment. Withhold ALUNBRIG for new or worsening respiratory symptoms and promptly evaluate for ILD/pneumonitis. Upon recovery, either dose reduce or permanently discontinue ALUNBRIG.

• Hypertension: monitor blood pressure after 2 weeks and then at least monthly during treatment. For severe hypertension, withhold ALUNBRIG, then dose reduce or permanently discontinue.

(Figure X. Main complications of persistent hypertension

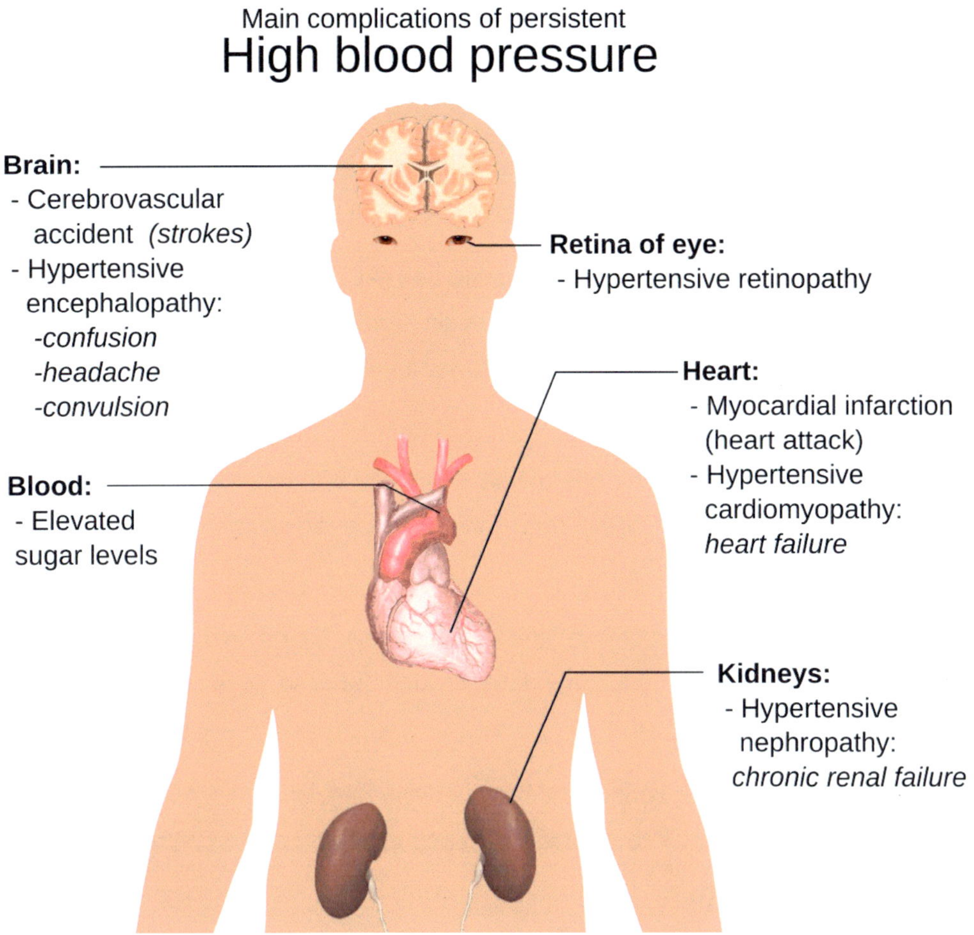

This image is by Mikael Häggström. Public Domain, https://commons.wikimedia.org/w/index.php?curid=5678966; https://en.wikipedia.org/wiki/Hypertension#/media/File:Main_complications_of_persistent_high_blood_pressure.svg. the copyright holder of this work, release this work into the public domain. No changes were made to this image).

Duration of intracranial response was measured from date of first intracranial response until intracranial disease progression (new lesions, intracranial target lesion diameter growth ≥20% from nadir, or unequivocal progression of intracranial nontarget lesions) or death.

• Bradycardia: monitor heart rate and blood pressure regularly during treatment. If symptomatic, withhold ALUNBRIG, then dose reduce or permanently discontinue.

• Visual Disturbance: advise patients to report visual symptoms. Withhold ALUNBRIG and obtain ophthalmologic evaluation, then dose reduce or permanently discontinue ALUNBRIG.

• Creatine phosphokinase (CPK) elevation: monitor CPK levels regularly during treatment. Based on the severity and with muscle pain or weakness, withhold ALUNBRIG, then resume or reduce dose.

• Pancreatic enzymes elevation: monitor lipase and amylase levels regularly during treatment. Based on the severity, withhold ALUNBRIG, then resume or reduce dose.

• Hepatotoxicity: monitor alanine aminotransferase (ALT), aspartate aminotransferase (AST) and total bilirubin levels regularly during treatment. Based on severity, withhold dose, then resume at lower level.

• Hyperglycemia: assess fasting serum glucose prior to starting ALUNBRIG and regularly during treatment. If not adequately controlled with optimal medical management, withhold ALUNBRIG, then consider dose reduction or permanently discontinue, based on severity.

• Photosensitivity: advise patients to limit sun exposure. Based on severity withhold ALUNBRIG, then resume at the same dose, reduce the dose, or permanently discontinue.

• Embryo-fetal toxicity: can cause fetal harm. Advise females of reproductive potential of the potential risk to a fetus and to use effective contraception.

ADVERSE REACTIONS

The most common adverse reactions (≥25%) with ALUNBRIG were diarrhea, fatigue, nausea, rash, cough, myalgia, headache, hypertension, vomiting, and dyspnea. To report SUSPECTED ADVERSE REACTIONS, contact Takeda Pharmaceuticals at 1-844-217-6468 or FDA at 1-800-FDA-1088 or www.fda.gov/medwatch.

DRUG INTERACTIONS

• CYP3A Inhibitors: avoid coadministration of ALUNBRIG with strong or moderate CYP3A inhibitors. If coadministration of a strong or moderate CYP3A inhibitor is unavoidable, reduce the dose of ALUNBRIG. *(Potent inhibitors of CYP3A4 include clarithromycin, erythromycin, diltiazem, itraconazole, ketoconazole, ritonavir, verapamil, goldenseal and grapefruit).*

• CYP3A Inducers: avoid coadministration of ALUNBRIG with strong or moderate CYP3A inducers. *(see list of strong CYP3A inducers in section on Tagrisso)*

If coadministration of a moderate CYP3A inducer is unavoidable, increase the dose of ALUNBRIG.

USE IN SPECIFIC POPULATIONS

- Hepatic Impairment: Reduce the dose of ALUNBRIG for patients with severe hepatic impairment.
- Renal Impairment: reduce the dose of ALUNBRIG for patients with severe renal impairment.
- Lactation: advise not to breastfeed.

DESCRIPTION

Mechanism of action

Brigatinib is a tyrosine kinase inhibitor (TKI) with in vitro activity at clinically achievable concentrations against multiple kinases including ALK, ROS1, insulin-like growth factor-1 receptor (IGF-1R), and FLT-3 as well as EGFR deletion and point mutations. Brigatinib inhibited autophosphorylation of ALK and ALK-mediated phosphorylation of the downstream signalling proteins STAT3, AKT, ERK1/2, and S6 in in vitro and in vivo assays. Brigatinib also inhibited the in vitro proliferation of cell lines expressing EML4-ALK and NPM-ALK fusion proteins and demonstrated dose-dependent inhibition of EML4-ALK-positive NSCLC xenograft growth in mice. At clinically achievable concentrations (≤500 nM), brigatinib inhibited the in vitro viability of cells expressing EML4-ALK and 17 mutant forms associated with resistance to ALK inhibitors including crizotinib, as well as EGFR-Del (E746-A750), ROS1-L2026M, FLT3-F691L, and FLT3-D835Y. Brigatinib exhibited in vivo antitumor activity against 4 mutant forms of EML4-ALK, including G1202R and L1196M mutants identified in NSCLC tumors in patients who have progressed on crizotinib. Brigatinib also reduced tumor burden and prolonged survival in mice implanted intracranially with an ALK-driven tumor cell line. 12.2 Pharmacodynamics

CLINICAL STUDIES

1. TKI-naïve advanced ALK-positive NSCLC (ALTA 1L Study)

The efficacy of ALUNBRIG was demonstrated in a randomized (1:1), open-label, multicenter trial (ALTA 1L, NCT02737501) in adult patients with advanced ALK-positive NSCLC who had not previously received an ALK-targeted therapy. The study required patients to have an ALK rearrangement based on a local standard of care testing. Eligible patients were allowed to have up to 1 prior regimen of chemotherapy in the locally advanced or metastatic setting and were required to have an ECOG Performance Status of 0-2. Neurologically stable patients with treated or untreated central nervous system (CNS) metastases, including leptomeningeal metastases, were eligible. Patients with a history of interstitial lung disease, drug-related pneumonitis, or radiation pneumonitis were excluded.

The major efficacy outcome measure was progression-free survival (PFS) as evaluated by a Blinded Independent Review Committee (BIRC) according to Response Evaluation Criteria in Solid Tumors (RECIST v1.1). Additional efficacy outcome measures included confirmed overall response rate (ORR), duration of response (DOR), intracranial ORR, and intracranial DOR as evaluated by BIRC, and overall survival (OS). A total of 275 patients were randomized to receive ALUNBRIG 180 mg orally once daily with a 7-day lead-in at 90 mg once daily (n = 137) or crizotinib 250 mg orally twice daily (n = 138). Of the 275 enrolled patients, 239 had positive results using the companion diagnostic test, the Vysis ALK Break Apart FISH Probe Kit; central results were negative for 20 patients and unavailable for 16 patients. Crossover from the crizotinib arm to the ALUNBRIG arm was permitted following disease progression. Randomization was stratified by CNS metastases (present vs absent) and prior chemotherapy use for locally advanced or metastatic disease (yes, no). Baseline demographic characteristics of the overall study population were: median age 59 years (range: 27 to 89, 32% 65 and over), 59% White and 39% Asian, 55% female, 39% ECOG PS 0 and 56% ECOG PS 1, and 58% never smokers. The disease characteristics of the overall study population were: 93% with Stage IV disease; 27% received chemotherapy in the locally advanced or metastatic setting; 14% had received CNS radiation; 31% had bone metastases; and 20% had liver metastases. CNS metastases were present in 35% (n = 96) of patients; 41 of those patients had measurable CNS lesions. ALTA 1L demonstrated a statistically significant improvement in PFS by BIRC.

At the final analysis of overall survival, conducted approximately 3 years after the last patient enrolled, there were 92 deaths (33% of all patients) including 41 deaths on the ALUNBRIG arm and 51 deaths on the crizotinib arm; median OS was not reached on either arm. Duration of intracranial response was measured from date of first intracranial response until intracranial disease progression (new lesions, intracranial target lesion diameter growth ≥20% from nadir, or unequivocal progression of intracranial nontarget lesions) or death.

2. ALK-positive advanced or metastatic NSCLC previously treated with crizotinib

The efficacy of ALUNBERG was demonstrated in a two-arm, open-label, multicenter trial (ALTA, NCT02094573) in adult patients with locally advanced or metastatic ALK-positive non-small cell lung cancer (NSCLC) who had progressed on crizotinib. The study required patients to have a documented ALK rearrangement based on an FDA-approved test or a different test with adequate archival tissue to confirm ALK arrangement by the Vysis® ALK Break-Apart fluorescence in situ hybridization (FISH) Probe Kit test. Key eligibility criteria included an ECOG Performance Status of 0-2 and progression on crizotinib. Neurologically stable patients with central nervous system (CNS) metastases were permitted to enroll. Patients with a history of interstitial lung disease or drug-related pneumonitis or who had received crizotinib within 3 days of the first dose of brigatinib were excluded. The major efficacy outcome measure was confirmed overall response rate (ORR) according to Response Evaluation Criteria in Solid Tumors (RECIST v1.1) as evaluated by an Independent Review Committee (IRC). Additional efficacy outcome measures included Investigator-assessed ORR, duration of response (DOR), intracranial ORR, and intracranial DOR. A total of 222 patients were randomized to receive ALUNBRIG either 90 mg once daily (90 mg arm; n = 112) or 180 mg once daily following a 7-day lead-in at 90 mg once daily (90→180 mg arm; n = 110). Randomization was stratified by CNS metastases (present vs absent) and best prior response to crizotinib (complete or partial response vs any other response/unevaluable). Baseline demographic characteristics of the overall study population were: median age 54 years (range: 18 to 82, 23% 65 and over), 67% White and 31% Asian, 57% female, 36% ECOG PS 0 and 57% ECOG PS 1, and 95% never or former smokers. The disease characteristics of the overall study population were: stage IV disease in 98%, adenocarcinoma histology in 97%, prior systemic chemotherapy in 74%, CNS metastases in 69% (61% had received prior CNS radiation), bone metastases in 39%, and liver metastases in 26% of patients.

Sixty-four percent of patients had an objective response to prior crizotinib. The median duration of follow-up was 8 months (range: 0.1 to 20.2).

Duration of intracranial response was measured from date of first intracranial response until intracranial disease progression (new lesions, intracranial target lesion diameter growth ≥20% from nadir, or unequivocal progression of intracranial nontarget lesions) or death.

(iii) LORLATINIB (LORBRENA)

HIGHLIGHTS OF PRESCRIBING INFORMATION These highlights do not include all the information needed to use LORBRENA safely and effectively. See full prescribing information for LORBRENA. LORBRENA® (lorlatinib) tablets, for oral use Initial U.S. Approval: 2018

INDICATIONS AND USAGE

LORBRENA is a kinase inhibitor indicated for the treatment of patients with anaplastic lymphoma kinase (ALK)-positive metastatic non-small cell lung cancer (NSCLC) whose disease has progressed on

- crizotinib and at least one other ALK inhibitor for metastatic disease; or
- alectinib as the first ALK inhibitor therapy for metastatic disease; or
- ceritinib as the first ALK inhibitor therapy for metastatic disease. This indication is approved under accelerated approval based on tumor response rate and duration of response. Continued approval for this indication may be contingent upon verification and description of clinical benefit in a confirmatory trial.

12.1 Mechanism of Action

Lorlatinib is a kinase inhibitor with in vitro activity against ALK and ROS1 as well as TYK1, FER, FPS, TRKA, TRKB, TRKC, FAK, FAK2, and ACK. Lorlatinib demonstrated in vitro activity against multiple mutant forms of the ALK enzyme, including some mutations detected in tumors at the time of disease progression on crizotinib and other ALK inhibitors. In mice subcutaneously implanted with tumors harboring EML4 fusions with either ALK variant 1 or ALK mutations, including the G1202R and I1171T mutations detected in tumors at the time of disease progression on ALK inhibitors, administration of lorlatinib resulted in antitumor activity. Lorlatinib also demonstrated anti-tumor activity and prolonged survival in mice implanted intracranially with EML4-ALK-driven tumor cell lines. The overall antitumor activity of lorlatinib in in vivo models was dose-dependent and correlated with inhibition of ALK phosphorylation.

DOSAGE AND ADMINISTRATION

The recommended dosage is 100 mg orally once daily.

DOSAGE FORMS AND STRENGTHS

Tablets: 25 mg or 100 mg.

CONTRAINDICATIONS

Concomitant use with strong CYP3A inducers *(see list of strong CYA3P inducers in section on Tagrisso)*

WARNINGS AND PRECAUTIONS

• Risk of serious hepatotoxicity with concomitant use of strong CYP3A inducers: discontinue strong CYP3A inducers for 3 plasma half-lives of the strong CYP3A inducer prior to initiating LORBRENA

• Central nervous system (CNS) effects

CNS effects include seizures, hallucinations and changes in cognitive function, mood (including suicidal ideation), speech, mental status, and sleep. Withhold and resume LORBRENA at same or reduced dose or permanently discontinue LORBRENA based on severity.

• Hyperlipidemia: initiate or increase the dose of lipid-lowering agents. Withhold and resume LORBRENA at same or reduced dose based on severity.

• Atrioventricular block

Withhold and resume LORBRENA at same or reduced dose based on severity.

(Figure X. ECG Leads I and II demonstrating complete AV block. Note that the P waves are not related to the QRS complexes (PP interval and QRS interval both constant), demonstrating that the atria are electrically disconnected from the ventricles. The QRS complexes represent an escape rhythm arising from the ventricle).

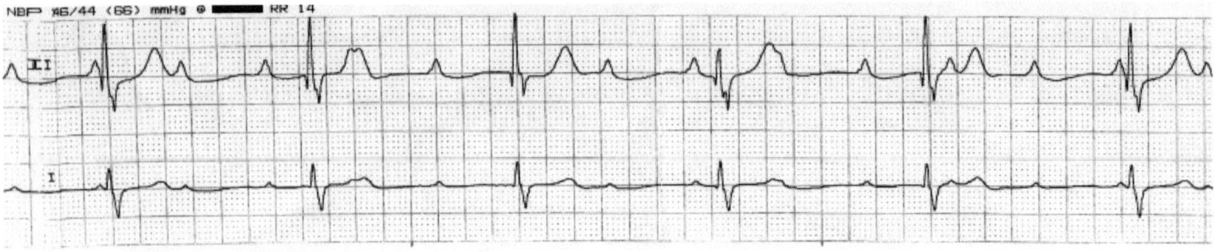

(This image is by MoodyGroove at English Wikipedia - Own work, Public Domain, https://commons.wikimedia.org/w/index.php?curid=18055698; https://en.wikipedia.org/wiki/Third-degree_atrioventricular_block#/media/File:Rhythm_strip_showing_third_degree_heart_block.jpg. This work has been released into the public domain by its author, MoodyGroove at English Wikipedia. No changes were made to this image).

• Interstitial lung disease/pneumonitis

Immediately withhold LORBRENA in patients with suspected ILD/pneumonitis. Permanently discontinue LORBRENA for treatment-related ILD/pneumonitis of any severity.

• Embryo-fetal toxicity:

can cause fetal harm. Advise females of reproductive potential of the potential risk to a fetus. Advise males and females of reproductive potential to use an effective non-hormonal method of contraception.

ADVERSE REACTIONS

Most common adverse reactions (incidence ≥20%) are edema, peripheral neuropathy, cognitive effects, dyspnea, fatigue, weight gain, arthralgia, mood effects, and diarrhea.To report SUSPECTED ADVERSE REACTIONS, contact Pfizer, Inc. at 1-800-438-1985 or www.pfizer.com or FDA at 1-800-FDA-1088 or www.fda.gov/medwatch.

DRUG INTERACTIONS

- CYP3A inducers: contraindicated with strong CYP3A inducers *(see list of strong CYP3A4 inducers in section on Tagrisso)*. Avoid concomitant use with moderate CYP3A inducers.

- CYP3A inhibitors: avoid concomitant use with strong CYP3A inhibitors; reduce LORBRENA dose if concomitant use cannot be avoided. *(Potent inhibitors of CYP3A4 include clarithromycin, erythromycin, diltiazem, itraconazole, ketoconazole, ritonavir, verapamil, goldenseal and grapefruit).*

- CYP3A substrates: avoid concomitant use with CYP3A substrates, where minimal concentration changes may lead to serious therapeutic failures. *CYP3A substrates include clarithromycin. diltiazem. erythromycin. fluconazole. grapefruit juice, itraconazole, ketoconazole, posaconazole. voriconazole and verapamil.*

USE IN SPECIFIC POPULATIONS

Lactation: advise not to breastfeed.

12.1 Mechanism of Action

Lorlatinib is a kinase inhibitor with in vitro activity against ALK and ROS1 as well as TYK1, FER, FPS, TRKA, TRKB, TRKC, FAK, FAK2, and ACK. Lorlatinib demonstrated in vitro activity against multiple mutant forms of the ALK enzyme, including some mutations detected in tumors at the time of disease progression on crizotinib and other ALK inhibitors. In mice subcutaneously implanted with tumors harboring EML4 fusions with either ALK variant 1 or ALK mutations, including the G1202R and I1171T mutations detected in tumors at the time of disease progression on ALK inhibitors, administration of lorlatinib resulted in antitumor activity. Lorlatinib also demonstrated anti-tumor activity and prolonged survival in mice implanted intracranially with EML4-ALK-driven tumor cell lines. The overall antitumor activity of lorlatinib in in vivo models was dose-dependent and correlated with inhibition of ALK phosphorylation.

14. CLINICAL STUDIES

14.1 ALK-Positive Metastatic NSCLC Previously Treated with an ALK Kinase Inhibitor The efficacy of LORBRENA was demonstrated in a subgroup of patients with ALK-positive metastatic non-small cell lung cancer (NSCLC) previously treated with one or more ALK kinase inhibitors who were enrolled in a non-randomized, dose-ranging and activity-estimating, multi-cohort, multicenter study (Study B7461001; NCT01970865). Patients included in this subgroup were required to have metastatic disease with at least 1 measurable target lesion according to Response Evaluation Criteria in Solid Tumors (RECIST) version 1.1 (v1.1), ECOG performance status of 0 to 2, and documented ALK rearrangement in tumor tissue as determined by fluorescence in situ hybridization (FISH) assay or by Immunohistochemistry (IHC), and received LORBRENA 100 mg orally once daily. Patients with asymptomatic CNS metastases, including patients with stable or decreasing steroid use within 2 weeks prior to study entry, were eligible. Patients with severe, acute, or chronic psychiatric conditions including suicidal ideation or behavior were excluded. In addition, for patients with ALK-positive metastatic NSCLC, the extent and type of prior treatment was specified for each individual cohort (see Table 4). The major efficacy outcome measures were overall response rate (ORR) and intracranial ORR, according to RECIST v1.1, as assessed by Independent Central Review (ICR) committee. Data were pooled across all subgroups listed in Table 4. Additional efficacy outcome measures included duration of response (DOR), and intracranial DOR. A total of 215 patients were enrolled across the subgroups in Table 4. The distribution of patients by type and extent of prior therapy is provided in Table 4. The demographic characteristics across all 215 patients were: 59% female, 51% White, 34% Asian, and the median age was 53 years (29 to 85 years) with 18% of patients ≥65 years. The ECOG performance status at baseline was 0 or 1 in 96% of patients. All patients had metastatic disease and 95% had adenocarcinoma. Brain metastases as identified by ICR were present in 69% of patients; of these, 60% had received prior radiation to the brain and 60% (n=89) had measurable disease per ICR.

An assessment of intracranial ORR and the duration of response for CNS metastases in the subgroup of 89 patients in Study B7461001 with baseline measurable lesions in the CNS according to RECIST v1.1 was performed. Of these, 56 (63%) patients received prior brain radiation, including 42 patients (47%) who completed brain radiation treatment at least 6 months before starting treatment with LORBRENA.

Response rate 60% (95% CI 49, 71)

Complete response 21%

Partial response 38%

Duration of response (median, months) 19.5 (95% CI:12.4, not reached)

In exploratory analyses conducted in subgroups defined by prior therapy, the response rates to LORBRENA were:

- ORR = 39% (95% CI: 30, 48) in 119 patients who received crizotinib and at least one other ALK inhibitor, with or without prior chemotherapy
- ORR = 31% (95% CI: 9, 61) in 13 patients who received alectinib as their only ALK inhibitor, with or without prior chemotherapy
- ORR = 46% (95% CI: 19, 75) in 13 patients who received ceritinib as their only ALK inhibitor, with or without prior chemotherapy

8. Conclusions

Imatinib, the first protein kinase developed and approved by the FDA for therapeutic use in chronic myeloid leukemia, revolutionized treatment for this disease. However, resistance to it developed in some patients and subsequent generations of TKIs have been developed to counter this. Allogeneic hematopoietic stem cell transplantation remains the only curative treatment for it, but has a treatnment-related mortality of 20 – 30%.

The TKIs now in use for NSCLC have likewise made an astonishing improvement in the outcome of NSCLC, but are not curative. However, they, and another new class of drugs – the checkpoint inhibitors - have shown that progress can, and is being , made in this disease, which has been so difficult to treat until the introduction of these new medications.

ABBREVIATIONS USED

Abbreviations used (other than those explained in the FDA Highlights of Prescribing and the FDA Full Prescribing Information) are listed below. This list includes abbreviations used in other books in the series Medicine 2020 and the series Modern Medicine.

AC, adriamycin and cyclophosphamide (combination chemotherapy)

ACE, angiotensin-converting-enzyme

ADC, antibody-drug conjugate

ADCC, antibody-dependent cellular cytotoxicity

ADCC, antibody directed enzyme prodrug therapy

AGEP, acute generalized exanthematous pustulosis

AI, aromatase inhibitor

ALK, anaplastic lymphoma kinase

ALL, acute lymphoblastic leukemia

ALT, alanine aminotransferase

AML, acute myeloid leukemia

aPTT, activated partial thromboplastin time

ARR, administration-related reaction

AS, adverse reaction

AS, ankylosing spondylitis

ASCT, autologous stem cell transplant

AST, aspartate aminotransferase

ATA, anti-therapeutic antibody

ATM, ataxia telangiectasia mutated (gene)

AUC, Area Under the Concentration – time curve

AUC (0-inf): AUC curve to infinite time. As we cannot get the assays to go to infinity, we have to extrapolate to infinity. This can be calculated from the AUC(0-t) by the addition of a constant (Clast/λz), where Clast is the last observed quantifiable concentration and λz is the terminal phase rate constant.

BCG, Bacille Calmain-Guerin

BCMA, B cell maturation antigen

BCR-ABL, breakpoint cluster region/Abelson

BCRP, breast cancer resistance protein

b DMARD, biologic disease-modifying anti-rheumatic drug

BRACA1, breast cancer susceptibility gene 1

BTK, Bruton's tyrosine kinase

CAT, cyclophosphamide, adriamycin and taxane (combination chemotherapy)

CDC, complement-dependent cytotoxicity

CDK, cyclin-dependent kinase

C-G, Cockoft-Gault (formula)

cHL, classical Hodgkin Lymphoma

CINV, chemotherapy-induced nausea and vomiting

CIS, carcinoma in situ

CLL, chronic lymphocytic leukemia

Clcr, creatinine clearance rate

CMF, cyclophosphamide, methotrexate, and fluorouracil (combination chemotherapy

CML, chronic myelogenous leukemia (also known as chronic myeloid leukemia)

CPS, combine positive score

CR, complete remission

CRC, colorectal carcinoma

CRISPR, clustered regulatory interspaced short palindromic repeats

CRS, cytokine release syndrome

CS, cytokine storm

csDMARD, synthetic disease-modifying anti-rheumatic drug

CSF1R, colony-stimulating factor receptor 1

CT, computed tomography

CTCAE, Common Terminology Criteria for Adverse Events

CVVHD, continuous veno-venous hemodialysis

DBCL, diffuse B cell lymphoma

DCIS, ductal carcinoma in situ

DFS, disease-free survival

dMMR, deficient mismatch repair

DLBCL, diffuse large B cell lymphoma

DMSO, dimethyl sulfoxide

DPP4, dipeptidyl peptidase-4

DRESS, drug reaction with eosinophilia and systemic symptoms. DRESS syndrome is classified as one form of severe cutaneous adverse reactions (SCARs). In addition to DRESS, SCARs includes four other drug-induced skin reactions, the Stevens–Johnson syndrome (SJS); Toxic epidermal necrolysis (TEN), Stevens–Johnson/toxic epidermal necrolysis overlap syndrome (SJS/TEN)

EBC, early breast cancer

ECG or EKG, electrocardiogram

EFS, event-free durvival

EGF, epidermal growth factor

EGFR, epidermal growth factor receptor

EN, erythema nodosum

ER, estrogen receptor

ET, endocrine therapy

ErbB, derived from erythroblastic leukemia viral oncogene

FBG, fasting blood glucose

FEC, fluorouracil, epirubicin and cyclophosphamide (combination chemotherapy)

FGF, fibroblast growth factor

FGFR, fibroblast growth factor receptor

FISH, fluorescence in situ hybridization

FKBP12/mTOR, FK Binding Protein-12/mammalian target of rapamycin

Flt3, fms like tyrosine kinase 3

FPG, fasting plams glucose

FSH, follicle-stimulating hormone

FU, fluouracil

gBRCAm, BRCA mutated

GBS, Guillain-Barré Syndrome

G-CSF, granulocyte colony-stimulating factor

GD, gestational day

GI, gastro-intestinal

GIST, gastrointestinal stromal tumor

GFR, glomerular filtration rate

GMR, geometric mean ratio

GVHD, graft-versus-host disease

HBV, hepatitis B

HCC, hepatocellular carcinoma

HCV, hepatitis C

HER, human epidermal receptor

HER2, human epidermal growth factor receptor 2

HIV, human immune deficiency virus

HNSCC, head and neck squamous carcinoma

HR, hormone receptor

HRR, homologous recombination repair

HSCT, hematopoietic stem cell transplant

JAK, Janus kinase

KLIFS-3, kinase-ligand interaction fingerprint and structure residue-3

IAP, intra-abdominal pressure

IBC, inflammatory breast cancer

IC, immune cell

ICANS, immune effector cell–associated neurotoxicity syndrome

IFN, interferon

IL, interleukin

ILD, interstitial lung disease

ILN, interstitial lung disease

iNHL, indolent non-Hodgkin lymphoma

IRIS, immune reconstitution inflammatory syndrome

IRR, infusion-related reaction

ITAM, immunoreceptor tyrosine-based activation motif

ITP, idiopathic thrombocytopenic purpura

LBCL, large B cell lymphoma

LCIS, lobular carcinoma in situ

LFT, liver function test

LH, luteinizing hormone

LLN, lower limit of normal

LVEF, left ventricular ejection fraction

Mab, monoclonal antibody

MATE, multi-antimicrobial extrusion protein

MBC, metastatic breast cancer

MCC, Merkel cell carcinoma

mCRPC, metastatic castrate resistant prostate cancer

MEK, mitogen-activated protein kinase

MRI, magnetic resonance imaging

MSI-H, microsatellite instability – high

MUGA, multigated acquisition

NCI-CTC, National Cancer Institute – Clinical Toxicity Criteria

Nib, small i**n**h**ib**itory molecule

NMIBC, non-muscle invasive bladder cancer

NRH, nodular regenerative hyperplasia (of the liver)

NSCLC, non-small cell lung cancer

OHSS, ovarian hyperstimulation syndrome

OS, overall survival

PARP, poly(ADP-ribose) polymerase

PDGF, platelet-derived growth factor

PDGFR, platelet-derived growth factor receptor

PFS, progression-free survival

Ph+, Philadelphia chromosome positive

PI3K, phosphatidylinositol 3-kinase

PI3KA, phosphatidylinositol-4,5-bisphosphate 3-kinase catalytic subunit alpha

PJIA, polyarticular juvenile idiopathic arthritis in patients aged 2 years or older

PJP, *Pneumocystis jiroveci* pneumonia

PK, pharmacokinetic analysis

PKA, protein kinase A

PMBCL, primary mediastinal B cell lymphoma

PML, progressive multifocal leukoencephalopathy

PNET, progressive neuroendocrine tumor (of the pancreas)

PR, progesterone receptor

pRb, retinoblastoma protein

PsA, psoriatic arthritis

PsO, plaque psoriasis

RA, rheumatoid arthritis

RAF, rapidly accelerated fibrosarcoma

RCC, renal cell carcinoma

REMS, Risk Evaluation and Mitigation Strategy

RET, "rearranged during transfection”

ROCK, Rho-associated protein kinase

ROS, 'orphan' receptor tyrosine kinase

rb, retinoblastoma (gene or protein)

r/r, relapsed/refractory

scFv, single-chain Fv fragment

SCARS, severe cutaneous adverse reactions

SCLC, small cell lung cancer

SERD, selective estrogen receptor degrader

SEGA, subependymal giant cell astrocytoma

SIRS, systemic inflammatory response syndrome

SLAM, signalling lymphocytic activation molecule family (CD319)

SJS, Stevens–Johnson syndrome

SLL, small lymphocytic lymphoma

SYK, spleen tyrosine kinase

SWFI, sterile water for injection

TALEN, transcription activator-like effector nuclease

TBC, tuberose sclerosid complex

TCH, docetaxel, carboplatin, and trastuzumab (combination chemotherapy)

TCR, T cell receptor

TEN, toxic epidermal necrolysis

TNBC, triple negative breast cancer

TMB- high, tunor mutational burden - high

TNF, tumor necrosis factor

TRK, tropomyosin receptor kinase

ts DMARD, targeted synthetic disease-modifying anti-rheumatic drug

Tyk, tyrosine-protein kinase

UGT1A1, uridine diphosphate-glucuronosyl transferase 1A1

ULN, upper limit of normal

VEGF, vascular endothelial growth factor

VEGFR, vascular endothelial growth factor receptor